Shrewd Cooking, Clever Eating: Masterful Meals for Smart Taste Buds" A Recipe for Progress"

Steve S. Morris

Table of contents..

Introduction:

- **The Specialty of Cooking Clever and Eating Perfect:**

In the clamoring mood of current life, the appeal of cheap food and pre-bundled feasts frequently appears to be overwhelming.

The simplicity of requesting in or destroying a frozen supper can be enticing, however what we lose in comfort, we gain in the split the difference of our wellbeing.

Enter the phenomenal universe of "Cooking Canny and Eating Perfect" - a culinary excursion that reclassifies the craft of cooking and supporting your body, all while embracing the sheer delight of gastronomy.

- Culinary Insight:

Cooking astutely isn't only about following recipes. It's tied in with procuring culinary knowledge, the ability to grasp the standards and study of food.

From dominating the speculative chemistry of flavors to saddling the force of flavors, this book guides you to turn into a culinary researcher.

You'll figure out how to make dishes that are flavorful as well as refreshing, as you open the mysteries of adjusted nourishment and careful eating.

- The Flavor Experience:

Cooking is an undertaking that connects every one of your faculties, and "Cooking Insightful and Eating Perfect" welcomes you on an enthralling flavor campaign.

Every part entices your taste buds with assorted cooking styles and novel fixings.
With bit by bit directions and enticing visuals, you'll cook your direction through scrumptious recipes from around the world.

An excursion of taste investigation will change your kitchen into an energetic food studio.

- Empowering Extravagance:

Eating extraordinary doesn't mean keeping yourself the delights from getting food; it implies relishing them with a careful point of view.

You'll reveal the sensitive harmony among extravagance and sustenance as you dive into faultless pastry recipes and debauched at this point solid treats.

From tasty chocolate treats to smooth smoothies, you'll find the enchantment of satisfying your sweet tooth without undermining your prosperity.

- Culinary Innovativeness:

The kitchen is your material, and each dish is a potential chance to release your innovativeness. "Cooking Sharp and Eating Perfect" urges you to turn into a craftsman with your culinary manifestations.

Investigate food pairings, explore different avenues regarding surfaces, and hoist your dinners to creativity.

Whether you're a beginner or an accomplished cook, this book welcomes you to dream, develop, and rethink your culinary abilities.

- Eating Great, Living Great:

Cooking clever and eating extraordinary isn't just about the food on your plate. Embracing a way of life focuses on prosperity.

From feasible cooking pursuits to careful eating routines, you'll find what your decisions in the kitchen can decidedly mean for your wellbeing and the climate.

This book is your passage to a comprehensive and manageable way to deal with feeding yourself and the planet.

- A Connoisseur Excursion Is standing by:

In "Cooking Shrewd and Eating Perfect," each page is an encouragement to set out on a connoisseur venture where the objective is great wellbeing, enticing flavors, and culinary dominance.

This book rises above simple recipes; a way of thinking commends the insight of cooking and the craft of enjoying.

It's a specialty worth relishing in itself, a creation of culinary insight that guarantees a long period of extraordinary eating and healthy living.

Express farewell to the accommodation of convenient solutions and express welcome to the specialty of cooking insightful and eating perfect.

Plunge into the kitchen with enthusiasm, embrace the specialty of careful cooking, and relish the kinds of a better, more delectable life. Your culinary experience starts

Chapter 1:

1. Kitchen Fundamentals:

Where Culinary Experiences Start In the core of each and every home, the kitchen rules as the focal point of sustenance, imagination, and local area.

Kitchen Fundamentals

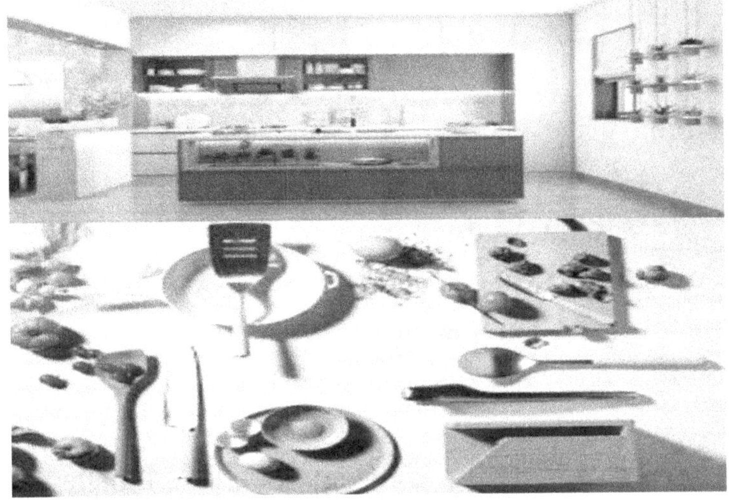

It is in this hallowed space that the enchantment of cooking unfurls, changing basic fixings into delicious dishes and long lasting recollections.

Welcome to the universe of "Kitchen Nuts and bolts," where we open the way to culinary dominance, and where each extraordinary gastronomic experience starts.

- The Culinary Material:

Consider your kitchen a fresh start anticipating your inventive touch. The fundamental kitchen rudiments are your range, fit to be changed into culinary show-stoppers.

This section establishes the groundwork for your cooking process by acquainting you with the instruments and hardware that will turn into your confided in partners.

From blades to cutting sheets, pots and dishes to spatulas, you'll find the unquestionable requirements and the pleasant to-haves for an exceptional kitchen.

- Blade Abilities: The Craft of Accuracy.

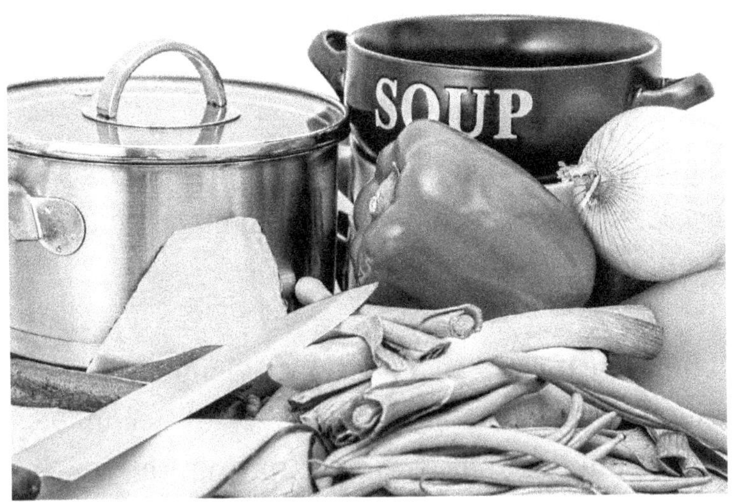

The blade is the culinary specialist's most devoted friend, and dominating blade abilities is the doorway to productive, exact, and pleasant cooking.

Kitchen Nuts and bolts, takes you through the basics of blade dealing, from picking the right cutting edge to culminating cutting, dicing, and slashing procedures.

You'll figure out how to change fixings from inconvenient to reasonable and make the cutting board your stage for culinary creativity.

- Cooking Procedures: The Language of the Kitchen.

Similarly as a painter learns brush strokes, a cook should become conversant in culinary methods.

This part is your manual for the language of the kitchen, showing you fundamental techniques like sautéing, simmering, braising, and that's only the tip of the iceberg.

With these abilities available to you, you'll acquire the capacity to adjust and make recipes with certainty, changing your fixings into agreeable, tasty dishes.

- Preparing and Flavor Building: The Ensemble of Taste.

At any point asked why eatery dishes burst with flavor? The response lies in the craft of preparing and flavor building.

"Kitchen Rudiments" acquaints you with the insider facts of making adjusted, enticing dishes. Figure out how to play with flavors, spices, acids, and umami-rich fixings, transforming your feasts into ensembles of taste that will leave your visitors hailing.

- The Storage room: A Universe of Fixings.

Your kitchen storage room is in excess of an assortment of fixings; it's a gold mine of culinary potential outcomes.

This section investigates the fundamentals of a very much supplied storeroom, from flavors and spices to grains, vegetables, and canned products.

Find the specialty of adjusting flavors and making dishes on the fly utilizing the wealth you have available.

- Food handling: Your Watchman in the Kitchen.

A genuine gourmet specialist is likewise a watchman of food handling.

"Kitchen Rudiments" takes you through the urgent standards of food handling, guaranteeing that your culinary manifestations enchant the sense of taste as well as safeguard your wellbeing and the prosperity of your friends and family.

* Association and Productivity:

The Way to Culinary Dominance Productivity
The kitchen is definitely not a blissful mishap; it's a consequence of smart association.

This part furnishes you with the standards of mise en place, the craft of setting up and arranging your kitchen before you begin cooking.

From preparing fixings to effective cleanup, you'll find how an efficient kitchen smoothes out your cooking cycle and upgrades your culinary encounters.

- Culinary Certainty: Your Visa to Investigation.

With kitchen nuts and bolts immovably close by, you'll be prepared to set out on a culinary excursion of investigation and inventiveness.

This section urges you to embrace your extraordinary culinary voice and move toward cooking with certainty and interest.

Whether you're reproducing family recipes or creating new dishes, your kitchen is currently a phase for your culinary creative mind.

- Conclusion:

The Delight of Cooking "Kitchen Fundamentals" isn't simply a manual; it's an encouragement to relish the delight of cooking.

It's a demonstration of the possibility that in the core of your home, basic fixings can become uncommon dinners.

With an exceptional kitchen, strong blade abilities, culinary procedures, and the craft of preparing, your culinary excursion has recently started.

Let "Kitchen Rudiments" be your aide as you leave on a deep rooted experience in the realm of flavors, fragrances, and important dinners.

Your kitchen is currently your material, and each dish you make is a work of art ready to be enjoyed.

2. Stacking Your Kitchen for Progress:

Where Culinary Dominance Starts.
Your kitchen is something other than a room where dinners are ready; it's the focal point of your culinary excursion, where you open your culinary potential.

Welcome to "Stacking Your Kitchen for Progress," the beginning stage of your way to culinary dominance.

This isn't just about loading your storage space; it's tied in with mixing your kitchen with the apparatuses, fixings, and motivation important for culinary advancement.

- An Exceptional Stockpile:

At the core of a well-working kitchen lies a munitions stockpile of instruments and hardware that can make your culinary dreams a reality.

"Stacking Your Kitchen for Progress" guides you through the fundamentals, guaranteeing your kitchen is prepared for progress.

From blades that cut with accuracy to the ideal cookware for your #1 dishes, you'll figure out how to pick and really focus on the apparatuses that will turn into your confided in colleagues in the kitchen.

- The Flexible Workhorse: Your Cutting Board.

A cutting board is something other than a piece of wood or plastic; it's the stage whereupon you make your culinary show-stoppers.

This section dives into the subtleties of picking the right cutting board, utilizing it accurately, and keeping up with its life span.

The cutting board isn't simply a kitchen fundamental; it's a material for your culinary innovativeness.

- The Ensemble of Flavor: Flavors and Flavors.

Flavors and flavors are the specialists in your culinary symphony, imbuing your dishes with notes of fervor and joy.

"Stacking Your Kitchen for Progress" acquaints you with the universe of flavors and flavors. You'll figure out how to assemble layers of flavor, make your unmistakable zest mixes, and lift your dishes to connoisseur levels.

- A Fair Storage room:

A very much supplied storage space is something beyond a stock of fixings; it's a wellspring of culinary motivation.

This section investigates the specialty of loading your storage space with a different exhibit of fixings, from grains and vegetables to oils, vinegars, and canned products.
With a fair storage room, you'll have the natural substances to explore and make unbounded.

- Culinary Certainty:

Certainty is the mysterious fixing to culinary achievement, and "Stacking Your Kitchen for Progress" sustains this fundamental quality.

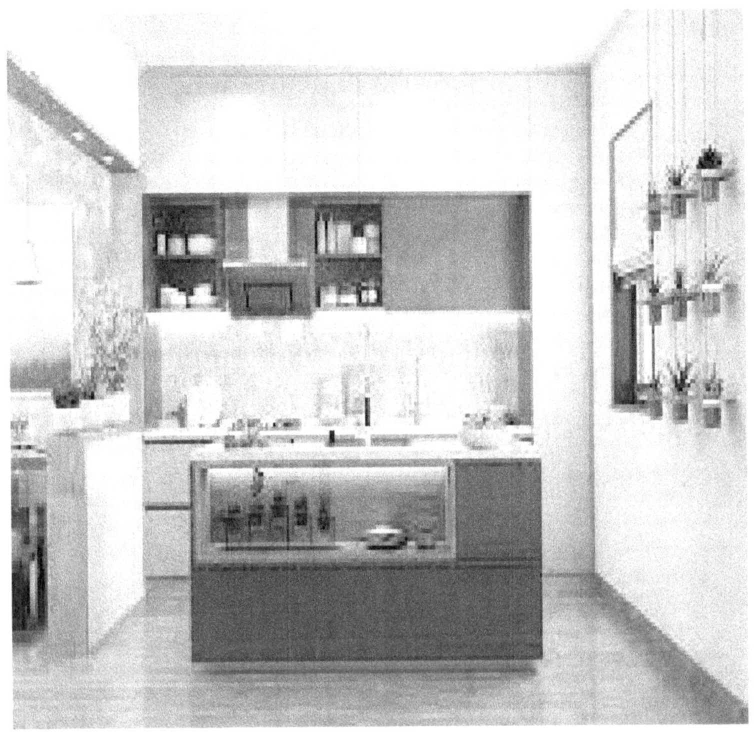

As you stock your kitchen and come out as comfortable with your devices, you'll feel a developing feeling of culinary strengthening.

This recently discovered certainty will encourage you to face challenges, try, and raise your culinary manifestations.

- Proficiency and Association:

Culinary authority isn't just about what you cook; it's additionally about how you cook. This section guides you through the standards of mise en place, the craft of arranging and setting up your fixings before you begin cooking.

An efficient kitchen guarantees effectiveness, diminishes pressure, and enables you to assume responsibility for your culinary excursion.

- Raise Your Faculties:

A dining experience for the eyes is a banquet for the spirit. "Stacking Your Kitchen for Progress" acquaints you with the craft of show and plating, telling you the best way to change your dishes into works of culinary workmanship.

Raise your culinary manifestations from simple food to visual show-stoppers that pleasure and rouse.

- Progress Past the Plate:

"Stacking Your Kitchen for Progress" isn't just about further developing your cooking abilities; it's an entryway to a more careful and charming way to deal with food.

As you embrace this excursion, you'll find that advancement in the kitchen rises above culinary abilities; it's a development of your relationship with food and the delight it brings to your life.

- Conclusion:

In the kitchen, progress is a ceaseless odyssey. "Stacking Your Kitchen for Progress" is your friend on this excursion, a manual for constant development, trial and error, and culinary creativity.

With your exceptional kitchen, an abundance of fixings, and newly discovered certainty, your culinary journey has started.

Allow it to be a demonstration of the surprising advancement that comes from embracing the craft of cooking.

Welcome to a reality where your kitchen isn't simply a room; it's the doorway to limitless culinary conceivable outcomes, and the stage for your culinary advancement and thriving.

3. Essential Instruments for Each Home Cook:

In the core of each and every home, the kitchen is a domain of boundless chance, where straightforward fixings are changed into culinary show-stoppers.

To set out on this culinary experience, furnishing your kitchen with crucial instruments is foremost.

Welcome to an existence where home cooks become culinary specialists, and where the right instruments lift your art.

- The Adaptable Gourmet expert's Blade:

In the event that the kitchen were a realm, the cook's blade would be the crown gem. This adaptable cutting edge is your trusted ally for all that from cutting to dicing, and cleaving to mincing.

Whether you're working with natural products, vegetables, meats, or spices, a quality gourmet specialist's blade is the groundwork of your culinary weapons store.
Keep it sharp, and you'll use a device of huge accuracy and power.

- The Paring Blade: Accuracy and Detail.

For fragile assignments that require artfulness, the paring blade ventures into the spotlight.

Stripping, managing, and complex cutting are where this minor edge sparkles.

It's your go-to apparatus for making delightfully decorated plates and it is wonderful to guarantee that everything about.

- The Utility Blade: A Moderate size Wonder.

Once in a while, a sharp edge that is bigger than a paring blade however more modest than a cook's blade is the best decision.

This is where the utility blade becomes possibly the most important factor. A flexible workhorse handles many errands, from cutting sandwiches to handling medium sized leafy foods.

- The Bread Blade: Cutting Flawlessness:

With regards to cutting bread, cake, and other sensitive heated merchandise, a bread blade's serrated edge is your dearest companion.

Its sharp teeth make spotless, exact cuts, guaranteeing that your cuts are however engaging as they may be tasty.

- Kitchen Shears: The Performing multiple tasks Wonder.

Kitchen shears resemble the Swiss Armed force blade of your kitchen. They can handle a heap of undertakings, from clipping spices and slicing poultry to opening bundling.

These convenient shears are an unquestionable necessity for any home cook.

- Cutting Sheets: Your Culinary Material.

A solid cutting board is the stage whereupon your culinary manifestations show signs of life. Select wooden or plastic sheets that are not difficult to spot and delicate on your blades.
Make sure to commit separate sheets for meats and vegetables to forestall cross-pollution.

- Blending Bowls: The Concordance of Fixings.

Blending bowls are the writers of your culinary orchestra. They come in different sizes to oblige anything from a little dressing to an enormous clump of batter.

Hardened steel and glass blending bowls are both superb decisions for their strength and simplicity of cleaning.

- Estimating Apparatuses: Accuracy Matters.

Baking and cooking request exactness, and that is where estimating apparatuses become vital.

Outfit your kitchen with a bunch of estimating cups and spoons for fluid and dry fixings, and a kitchen scale for exact estimations. Precise estimations guarantee steady and solid outcomes.

- Cookware:

An exceptional kitchen incorporates an assortment of cookware, like pans, skillets, pots, and baking dishes. Put resources into quality pieces that disseminate heat uniformly and can endure the afflictions of regular cooking. With the right cookware, you'll have the flexibility to prepare a great many recipes

- Utensils:

Utensils are the hands of your kitchen, and you'll require a determination of spatulas, spoons, utensils, and scoops to aid the specialty of cooking.

Every utensil has a particular reason, whether it's flipping, mixing, or serving, and together, they structure your culinary unit.

- Conclusion:

Each house cook's culinary excursion starts with the right devices. "Key Instruments for Each Home Cook" is your manual for furnishing your kitchen with the fundamentals.

These instruments are not simple apparatuses; they are your imaginative carries out, your confided in buddies on your journey into the universe of culinary innovativeness.

With the right instruments close by, your kitchen turns into a material for culinary imaginativeness, where the basic demonstration of cooking turns into a show-stopper ready to be made.

Embrace these basics, and leave on a culinary experience loaded up with vast conceivable outcomes and scrumptious revelations.

Chapter 2:

1. Wise Shopping:

In the clamoring walkways of supermarkets, the choices you have significantly affect your wellbeing, your wallet, and, surprisingly, the climate.

This is where the specialty of "Quick Shopping" becomes possibly the most important factor, an expertise that enables you to make wise, esteemed, cognizant, and mindful decisions in the realm of food.

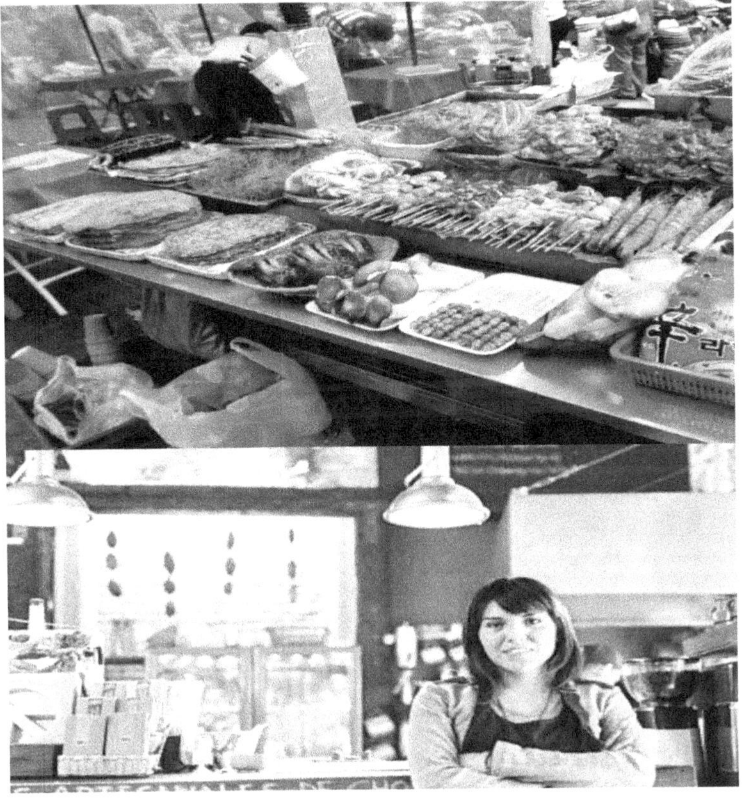

It's not just about exploring the walkways; it's tied in with changing the manner in which you approach shopping, carrying another degree of care to your truck.

- The Supermarket as Your Range:

Envision the supermarket as your culinary material, overflowing with a lively range of fixings. Canny shopping resembles choosing colors for a work of art; you pick your components with care and imagination.

From lively produce to storage room staples and enticing specialty things, everything in your truck adds to the show-stopper that is your dinner.

- Dominating Dinner Arranging:

Keen shopping starts before you even set foot in the store. Dinner arranging is your compass in this undertaking.

By framing your week after week feasts, you decrease food squander as well as guarantee you have the right fixings available, setting aside your time and cash.

This expertise changes your shopping list into an essential instrument that engages you to shop with reason.

- The Insight of Planning:

A quick customer doesn't just fill a truck; they stick to a financial plan. Monetary care is an essential component of quick shopping.

In light of an obvious spending plan, you can choose things that line up with your monetary objectives.

Whether it's picking store brands, contrasting costs, or searching for deals and limits, your spending plan fills in as your manual for shrewd and financially savvy staple decisions.

- Exploring the Border and Then some:

Have you at any point saw that the freshest, best, and most fundamental fixings in the store are many times tracked down along the edge?

The border houses the produce, dairy, meat, and new pastry shop segments, while the middle paths frequently contain handled and bundled food sources.

Smart shopping urges you to zero in on the border, where entire, natural, and supplement rich things rule. In any case, it likewise prepares you to explore the middle passageways nicely, choosing things that line up with your wholesome objectives.

- The Force of Names:

Wise shopping engages you to be a mark investigator. Understanding food names is fundamental for settling on informed decisions.

You'll figure out how to decipher wholesome names, fixing records, and different confirmations to guarantee that what you put in your truck lines up with your dietary inclinations and wellbeing targets.

- Purchase in Mass, Freeze, and Safeguard:

Purchasing in mass is a smart customer's clear-cut advantage. Besides the fact that it sets aside cash over the long haul, however it additionally limits bundling waste.

You'll likewise embrace the specialty of freezing and safeguarding, broadening the life expectancy of your food and decreasing food squander. This training isn't just financial plan amicable yet additionally naturally capable.

- Eco-Accommodating Decisions:

Adroit shopping isn't just about what's in your truck; it's likewise about the ecological effect of your decisions.

By choosing things with negligible bundling, purchasing privately obtained and reasonably developed produce, and picking eco-accommodating items, you add to a more feasible and mindful shopping for food experience.

- The Finish of Astute Shopping:

In the realm of canny shopping, your truck turns into an impression of your qualities, your wellbeing, cognizant choices, your monetary reasonability, and your obligation to the planet.

Quick shopping rises above simple excursions to the store; a lifestyle adjusts your decisions to your prosperity and everyone's benefit.

It changes shopping for food from an ordinary task into a significant demonstration of taking care of oneself and obligation.

The following time you explore the paths of your neighborhood supermarket, recollect that canny shopping isn't just about filling your truck; it's tied in with filling your existence with shrewdness, worth, and reason.

It's a work of art that engages you to pursue decisions that resonate with your qualities, changing your kitchen into a material where each feast is a show-stopper of wellbeing, economy, and manageability.

2. Overwhelming General store Course:

Exploring Shopping for food Like an Expert
The store: a maze of decisions, tones, and commitments. It's not difficult to lose all sense of direction in the labyrinth of choices, however with a clear cut technique and a sprinkle of keenness, you can overcome your general store

course   like   a   genius.

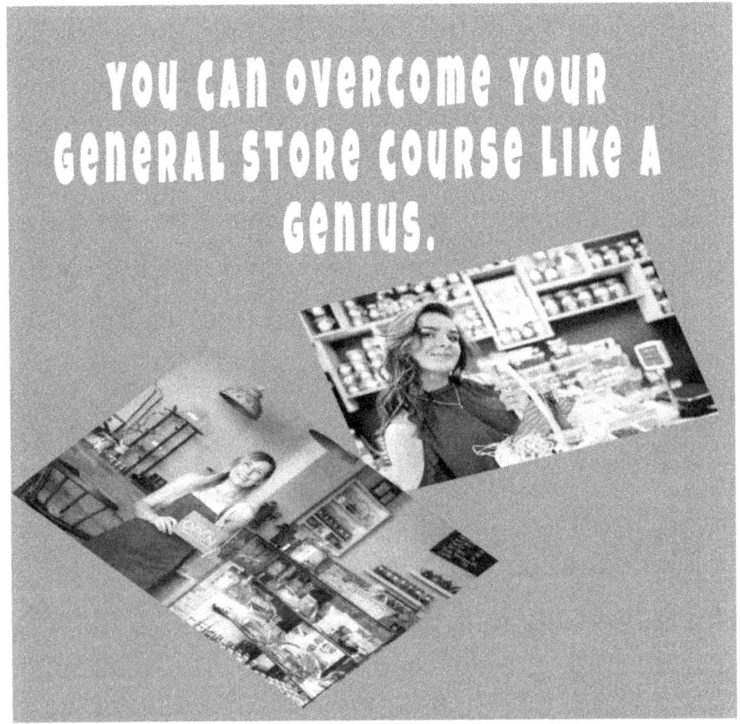

"Ruling Store Course" is your manual for turning into an expert of shopping for food, opening the mysteries of effectiveness, reserve funds, and solid decisions as you explore the paths like a carefully prepared customer.

- The Craft of Methodology:

Prior to venturing into the store, a shrewd customer has a blueprint. Plan your course by sorting out your rundown as per the store format.

Bunch things in classifications like produce, dairy, storeroom, and frozen, making your excursion more effective and less inclined to motivation buys.

- Key Shopping Times:

Pick your shopping times astutely.
Early mornings or non-weekend days frequently mean less groups and a more quiet climate, permitting you to shop all the more comfortably and settle on informed choices without the rush and interruptions.

- Subtle Shopping Rundown:

A good to go shopping list is your clear-cut advantage. Find an opportunity to make a rundown in view of your dinner plan and any family needs.

Stick to it, and you'll keep away from the appeal of pointless buys. Also, it's an eco-accommodating practice as it lessens food squander.

- Be careful with Spur of the moment purchases:

Stores are intended to entice you with tempting presentations and offers. Remain fixed on your rundown and your course, and try not to veer off from the arrangement except if you experience really helpful arrangements.

- Border Power:

The border of the grocery store is where you'll track down the freshest and best decisions. Begin your course by exploring the external edges, where you'll find produce, meats, dairy, and the bread kitchen area. These regions ordinarily house entire, natural, and supplement rich things.

- Focus Passageway Wariness:

While the border is your essential course, don't excuse the middle paths altogether. They contain staples like rice, pasta, canned merchandise, and other storage space fundamentals.

Utilize your rundown to direct you, guaranteeing you just enter these walkways for explicit requirements. Focus paths are additionally where you might track down flavors, toppings, and a few natural choices.

- Careful Meat Choice:

While visiting the meat area, be knowing. Decide on lean cuts, and consider buying bigger bits that can be isolated into more modest parts for freezing. It is much of the time more financially savvy to Purchase in mass.

- Dairy Choices:

Dairy decisions can overpower. Center around basics like milk, yogurt, and cheddar while watching out for deals and mass limits.

Furthermore, consider plant-based dairy options in the event that they line up with your dietary inclinations.

- Produce Pride:

In the produce area, center around occasional and nearby leafy foods. They're fresher as well as more spending plans are agreeable. Keep away from pre-cut or pre-bundled produce, which can be pricier.

- Smart Truck Association:

Your shopping basket isn't simply a vessel; it's an instrument for coordinating your course. Bunch things in your truck by class, keeping meat, dairy, and produce discrete.

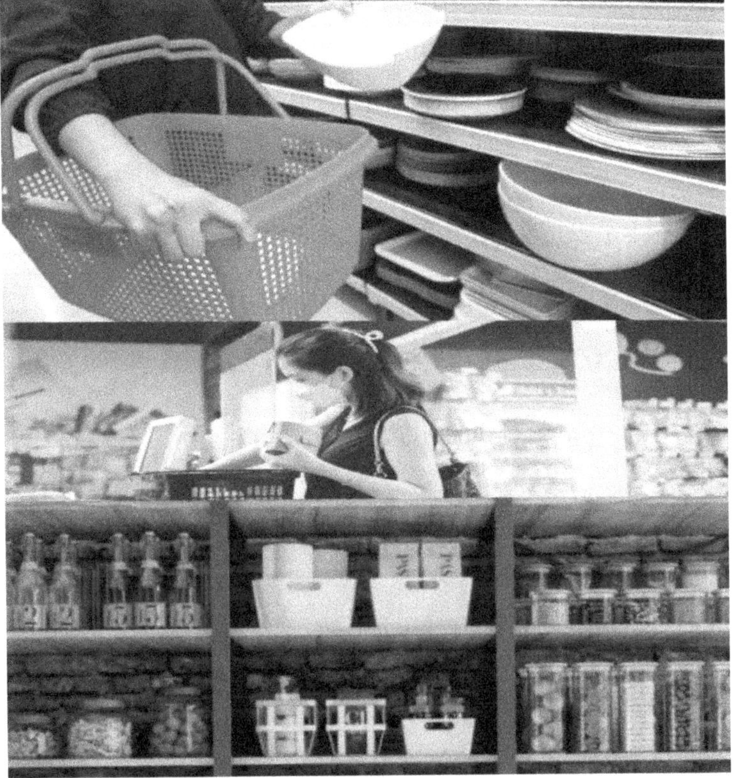

This aids during checkout as well as keeps fragile things from being crunched.

- Check for Limits:

Be cautious for limits, advancements, and deals all through your course. Frequently, deal things are situated toward the finish of paths or on independent showcases.

Notwithstanding, guarantee that these arrangements line up with your necessities and are things you'll really utilize.

- Careful Checkout:

The checkout is where motivation buys frequently strike. Keep on track and oppose the alarm call of enticing confections, magazines, and other last-minute things.

While pausing, twofold really look at your rundown to guarantee you haven't failed to remember anything fundamental.

Conclusion:

- Dominating the Course:

Ruling your grocery store course is more than proficient shopping; it's tied in with recapturing command over your decisions, your financial plan, and your prosperity.

This artistic expression guarantees you explore the walkways with reason, settling on informed choices that line up with your qualities and necessities.

As you embrace this training, you'll find that shopping for food isn't an errand yet a chance to communicate your culinary inclinations and values, changing your kitchen into a safe house of very much arranged, solid, and economical feasts.

In your excursion to ruling the store course, you become the overseer of your culinary story, guaranteeing that each fixing has a reason, each decision has meaning, and each feast turns into a delightful and careful experience.

3. Feast Arranging and Planning:

Picture this: giggling, fellowship, and the wonderful fragrance of an impeccably prepared feast drifting through the air.

This is the sorcery of banquet orchestrating and arranging. The craft of organizing remarkable culinary encounters doesn't simply occur by some coincidence; an expertise requires careful preparation, imagination, and a smidgen of sorcery.

"Feast Orchestrating and Arranging" is your manual for turning into a maestro of social events, changing dinners into remarkable recollections.

- The Specialty of Culinary Movement:

Each incredible banquet is a creation, and very much like a chief direction entertainers on a phase, you, as the host or leader, coordinate dishes on your table.

The menu is your content, the fixings, your cast, and the eating table. Talented movement guarantees that each dish has its impact in the orchestra of flavors, making an agreeable and noteworthy culinary experience.

- The Culinary Lyrics: Making Your Menu:

Your menu is the core of your culinary creation. Start by characterizing your topic and choosing dishes that line up with your vision.

Think about your visitors' dietary inclinations and limitations. As you plan your menu, ponder adjusting flavors, surfaces, and tones. Each dish ought to play a part to play, adding to the general concordance of the dinner.

- Practice: Recipe Testing.

Similarly as a play needs practice, your dishes require testing. Before the occasion, get ready and taste your picked recipes to guarantee they measure up to your assumptions. Change flavors, cooking times, and show until each dish sparkles.

- The Cast of Fixings: Shopping with Accuracy.

Feast orchestrating and arranging is incomplete without a shopping list. Make a rundown of the multitude of fixings you really want, taking consideration to stay away from superfluous additional items.

Plan your shopping great ahead of time, giving you an opportunity to look for the best fixings, limits, and arrangements.

Purchasing neighborhood and occasional produce can add an additional layer of newness to your dishes.

- The Troupe of Instruments: A Very much Supplied Kitchen.

A fruitful creation requires the right instruments. Guarantee your kitchen is outfitted with every one of the utensils and cookware expected to set up your picked dishes.

From pots and skillet to blades and cutting sheets, each device assumes a vital part in the culinary presentation.

- Projecting the Table: Table Setting and Stylistic layout.

Similarly as a scenery and stage configuration set the temperament for a dramatic presentation, your table setting and stylistic layout make the feeling for your banquet.

Pick your flatware, cloths, and focal points to line up with your subject and the air you need to summon. Insightful table setting upgrades the general eating experience.

- The Specialized Practice: Timing is Everything.

A fruitful dining experience is about immaculate timing. Plan your menu with conscious thought for cooking and serving times. Guarantee that you have a reasonable course of events for readiness and cooking.

A thoroughly examined plan limits pressure and guarantees that each dish shows up at the table at its pinnacle.

- The Orchestra of Administration:

Administration is an essential piece of your culinary presentation. Conclude whether you'll serve dishes family-style or independently.

On the off chance that you're having a bigger get-together, consider recruiting proficient servers or cooking administrations to guarantee consistent execution.

- The Stupendous Finale: Pastries and Desserts.

No banquet is finished without a show-halting pastry. Select sweet treats that reverberate with your subject and give a fitting end to your culinary excursion.

From intricate cakes to a choice of petits fours, sweets have an enduring impact on your visitors.

- Reprise: Making Enduring Recollections.

Feast organizing and arranging isn't just about the food; it's about the experience. Individual contacts, genuine motions, and smart take home gifts can transform a standard social occasion into an uncommon memory.

Consider how you can make your dining experience noteworthy for your visitors and make a reprise that waits in their psyches.

Conclusion:

- Your Culinary Magnum opus:

Feast orchestrating and arranging is a culinary work of art that changes dinners into vital encounters.

It's tied in with forming the ideal menu, assembling the right fixings, and coordinating each component of your social affair with accuracy.

Your culinary abilities are not just about cooking; they're tied in with making an environment, setting the stage, and creating enduring recollections.

As you become an expert of gala organizing and arranging, you step into the job of a culinary craftsman, winding around together the strings of flavor, environment, and experience to make a magnum opus that lives on in the hearts and recollections of your visitors.

Each social occasion turns into a presentation, each dish a star, and each second a heartfelt applause for your culinary virtuoso.

Chapter 3:

1. The Fundamentals of Cooking:

Building the Establishment for Culinary Dominance.

The Fundamentals of Cooking:

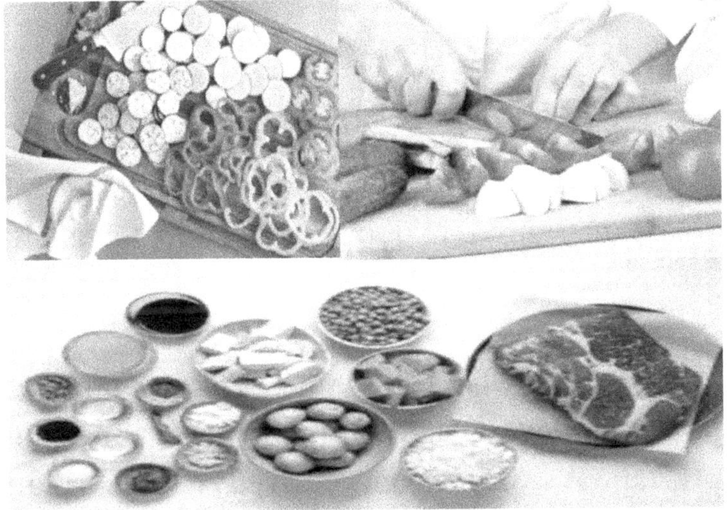

In the realm of culinary masterfulness, each gourmet expert, from the beginner home cook to the old pro, starts with the fundamentals of cooking.

These central standards are the structure blocks whereupon culinary dominance is built.

Whether you're stewing a pot of soup, burning a steak, or baking a soufflé, understanding the fundamentals of cooking is fundamental to hoist your dishes from common to phenomenal.

- Blade Abilities: The Specialty of Accuracy.

The kitchen's most fundamental apparatus is the blade. Blade abilities are the establishment whereupon any remaining culinary methods are assembled.

Whether it's cleaving, dicing, mincing, or julienning, excelling at accuracy with a blade is pivotal. A very much cleaved onion or an impeccably cut tomato can have a significant effect in the last dish.

- Heat Control: The Way to Dominance.

Heat control is an essential idea in cooking. It includes understanding how to control intensity to accomplish wanted results.

This implies knowing when to sauté at high intensity to singe a steak, and when to stew at low intensity to cajole flavors from a stew. It's tied in with accomplishing the right degree of doneness, delicacy, and caramelization in your fixings.

- Flavor Building: The Orchestra of Taste.

Culinary enchantment happens when you comprehend the specialty of flavor building. It's not just about preparing your dishes; it's tied in with layering and adjusting flavors to make an amicable entirety.

Fixings like spices, flavors, acids, and umami-rich parts assume urgent parts in this orchestra of taste.

Knowing when to add them and in what amounts can change your dishes into culinary works of art.

- The Culinary Trinity: Sauté, Broil, and Braise.

Sautéing, broiling, and braising are the major cooking procedures each hopeful gourmet specialist ought to dominate.

Sautéing includes speedy cooking in a limited quantity of oil, commonly utilized for vegetables or proteins.
Broiling is a dry-heat cooking technique that delightfully caramelizes fixings. Braising, then again, is the craft of slow-cooking fixings in a tasty fluid until delicate.

- The Study of Emulsification.

Emulsification is the most common way of blending two fixings that don't normally

consolidate, similar to oil and vinegar, to make a steady, velvety combination.
Salad dressings, mayonnaise, and vinaigrettes all depend on this procedure.

Dominating emulsification requires a comprehension of the science behind it, including the significance of gradually integrating one fixing into the other while whisking enthusiastically.

- Mise en Spot: The Craft of Planning.

Before the cooking starts, there's a fundamental step called mise en place, and that signifies "all things where they ought to be." It includes planning and coordinating every one of your fixings before you begin cooking.

This training saves time and guarantees that everything is all set, assisting you with remaining in charge of the cooking system.

- The Maillard Response: Flavor Speculative chemistry.

The Maillard response is a synthetic response between amino acids (proteins) and decreasing sugars that happens when food browns during cooking.

It's answerable for the complicated, appetizing flavors in food varieties like simmered meats, burned steaks, and toasted bread.
Understanding this response permits you to control the profundity of flavor in your dishes.

- Timing and Coordination: Accuracy Matters.

Cooking various parts of a feast all the while and organizing them to be prepared simultaneously is a workmanship.

Timing is basic to guarantee that everything is served hot and at its pinnacle. Being coordinated, having an unmistakable arrangement, and rehearsing your timing are vital components of culinary achievement.

- Neatness and Sanitation: The Foundation of Cooking.

A perfect and safe kitchen is the foundation of culinary creativity. This incorporates legitimate food dealing with, stockpiling, and cleanliness.

Security and tidiness not just safeguard you and your visitors from foodborne diseases yet in addition add to a consistent cooking experience.

Conclusion:

- The Way to Culinary Dominance:

The basics of cooking are the venturing stones on the way to culinary authority. They give the information and abilities important to transform crude fixings into tasty dishes.

While they might appear to be fundamental, they are the primary rules that permit you to release your imagination in the kitchen.

As you improve your blade abilities, ace intensity control, and comprehend the complexities of flavor, you'll change your cooking from simple food into an artistic expression.

The fundamentals of cooking are your compass, directing you on your culinary excursion, and your establishment, whereupon you'll construct your culinary inheritance.

2. Cooking Essentials:

Our involved fundamental cooking series is customized   for   fledglings.

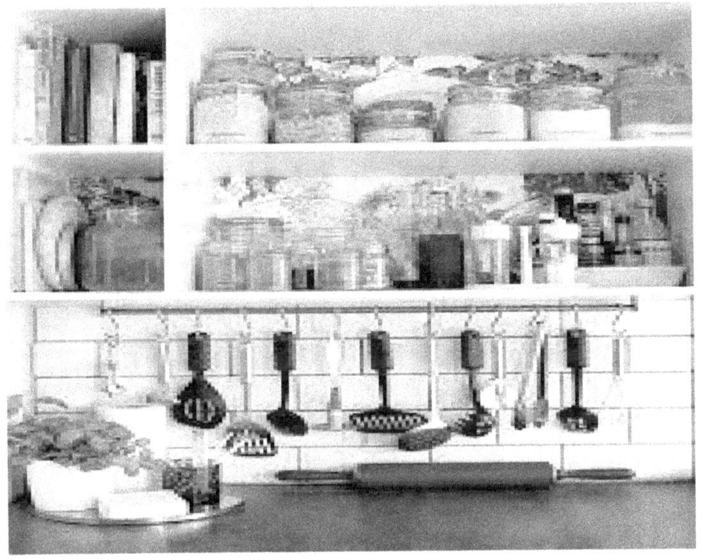

We'll direct you through total cooking nuts and bolts.

You'll learn fundamental culinary procedures through exemplary cooking strategies and connoisseur recipes!

We'll consider every contingency of the kitchen as we ace everything from proficient blade abilities to connoisseur introductions.
Gain proficiency with the essentials of cooking in this total active course.

• Cooking Fundamentals 1:

This series will give clear and brief recipes to ordinary cooking.
The class centers around straightforward procedures for effectively preparing dinners.

Figure out how to cook, dish singe, pan sear, make soups and basic sauces, and prepare without any preparation. Figure out how to plan superb dinners.

Blade Abilities and Vegetable Prep: Figure out how to assume command over your gourmet specialist's blade:

cutting, dicing and further developing your prep abilities, and comprehend which kitchen apparatuses are truly fundamental for the home cook. Figure out how to cut up an entire chicken.

Stocks, Soups and Sauces: Figure out how handcrafted stock makes all that in the kitchen taste better and engraving to memory the strategy for making impeccable soups.

Clear, stock based, puree, and cream soups; consommé; chowders; bisque; cold soups; soup decorating; soup administration.

Figure out how to make exemplary Sauces, present day sauces, and hand crafted fixings and use them in proficient style plating.

Pasta: Figure out how to cook and sauce ideal pasta with a portion of our home top picks.

Sauté: Sautéing is a fundamental cooking technique and appropriately sautéed proteins can be the base for a straightforward yet striking skillet sauce once you know a couple of key stunts. You'll attempt a few varieties.

- Cooking Basics 2

In view of the broadly famous book by Culinary specialist Samin Nosrat, every week we'll investigate one of these four essential components of cooking and how to best dominate that in your kitchen.

Salt, Fat, Corrosive, Intensity centers around the idea that dominating the utilization of four components will make any food heavenly:

salt, which improves flavor; fat, which conveys flavor and produces surface; corrosive, which adjusts flavor; and intensity, which at last decides the surface of food.

Salt: Find out about "Salt. It's crucial to all great cooking. It upgrades flavor and even makes food taste more such as itself.

So, salt rejuvenates food. Figure out how to utilize it well and your food will taste perfect."

Fat: Find out about "Fat. It's completely a supernatural occurrence. Fat is flavor. Fat is surface.

Fat adds its own remarkable flavor to a dish and it can enhance different flavors in a recipe.

Basically, fat makes food heavenly. Furthermore, perhaps the main thing any cook can learn is the manner by which to bridle its enchantment."

Corrosive: Find out about "Corrosive. It's the pucker in a lemon. It Is harsh in sharp cream.

The tart in cranberry sauce. It in a real sense makes mouths water. Corrosive lights up food and makes contrast.

Above all, corrosive does the totally important occupation of adjusting flavors, which makes it fundamental to preparing heavenly food."

- Heat: Find out about "Intensity.

It's the component of change.
Heat takes food from crude to cooked, out of shape to firm, pale to brilliant brown.
Sizzles, splatters, pops, steam, and fragrances are the consequences of applying intensity to food.

What's more, when you comprehend how intensity works, you can be certain that anything you cook will taste perfect."

- Cooking Fundamentals 3

This series will give clear and compact recipes to regular cooking.

The series centers around basic procedures for effectively preparing dinners.

Figure out how to broil, Poaching, Egg Cookery, Spice essentials. Figure out how to plan awesome dinners.

- Spice Essentials:

Spices are a tasty method for adding flavor to your food sources without adding additional calories! The class will assist you with matching different spices with your #1 food varieties to make sauces, plunges, fundamental dishes and even sweet!

- Broiling:

An extraordinary method for getting ready scrumptious courses for your loved ones.
Find the strategies that will ensure a positive outcome like clockwork.

We'll likewise talk about the various sorts of simmering skillet and whether vertical or level broiling is significant.

Barbecuing and Cooking: Everyone in the world loves to barbecue.
Whether you utilize a hibachi or an ex-55 gallon drum, everyone has their privileged insights.

We'll gain proficiency with a couple of expert methods, tips and recipes from us as we show you a definite fire ways of making your next grill a triumph!

Egg Cookery and Poaching: What appears to be so natural can end up being undeniably surprisingly troublesome.

This class will assist you with kicking your egg abilities up an indent. What is poaching?

A low-heat cooking strategy for meat and fish that will promise it stays wet and succulent.

3. Flavor Building and Preparing:

As a cook, it is my business to make paramount eating encounters and food that is remarkable.

Making dishes that truly wow the visitor is an innovative undertaking that includes every one of the faculties.

Ignoring even one sense will reduce the general effect and outcome of the dish. At the point when I make a dish, I think about its appearance.

Is it vivid, proportional with different shapes, adjusted among negative and positive spaces, all around planned, and for the most part appealing?

I ponder how sound could play into the dish with things like sizzle or crunch. Next I contemplate the dish's large fragrant profile that ought to be complex and alluring.

Then, at that point, I move to the mouth where I ponder the surface and taste.

An extraordinary dish joins various surfaces in various extents to keep the dish fascinating with each chomp.

With regards to taste, I consider how to consolidate every one of the five preferences — sweet, harsh, pungent, severe, and umami — in various sums to make a charming equilibrium of flavor.

Individuals are amazed to discover that every one of the five preferences would be able (and preferably ought to) fit into whatever number recipes as could be allowed.

The justification behind this is that we have different taste receptors for every one of our preferences. In this way, endeavoring to invigorate whatever number preferences as would be prudent makes a major taste impression and a more significant level of intricacy.

Be that as it may, how these preferences are consolidated and adjusted is the specialty of the dish, and there are a limitless assortment of mixes utilizing a large number of fixings.

Figuring out how to analyze various preferences for a recipe is fundamental for the inventive flow.

For example, bar-b-que sauces consolidate each of the five preferences for changing sums to accomplish different flavor profiles.

Pastries are dominatingly sweet and here and there harsh. Simultaneously, pastries utilize different preferences — yet in a foundation job. For example, chocolate, espresso, and caramel add unpleasant notes.

Salt in different batters or in chocolate arrangements is fundamental. Umami is progressively tracked down in sweets that consolidate bacon, prosciutto, or green tea.

- Noticeable Job for Umami:

Cooks today are progressively zeroing in on umami and making it a more unmistakable and thoroughly examined piece of their manifestations.

The explanation is straightforward. Umami contributes a base note that adds profundity of flavor and expands the exquisite (and tasty) character. There are two essential approaches to adding umami.

The first is using MSG, which is basically unadulterated umami.
The alternate way is using umami-rich fixings like miso, soy sauce, dried shiitake, ketchup, ocean growth, matured fish sauce, restored meats, very much matured cheeses, and so on.

When to utilize either procedure is an issue of the general impression you need. At the point when I use MSG, it is on the grounds that I need umami without different flavors.

At the point when I use umami-rich fixings, it is the point at which I need more umami and different flavors.

An investigation of the ramen recipe beneath gives a smart thought of how various fixings contribute various things to the last dish.

Chapter 4:

1. Quick and Easy Weeknight Blowouts:

Life's hurrying around can some of the time leave us longing for speedy and fulfilling arrangements, particularly with regards to

Quick and Easy
Weeknight Blowouts:

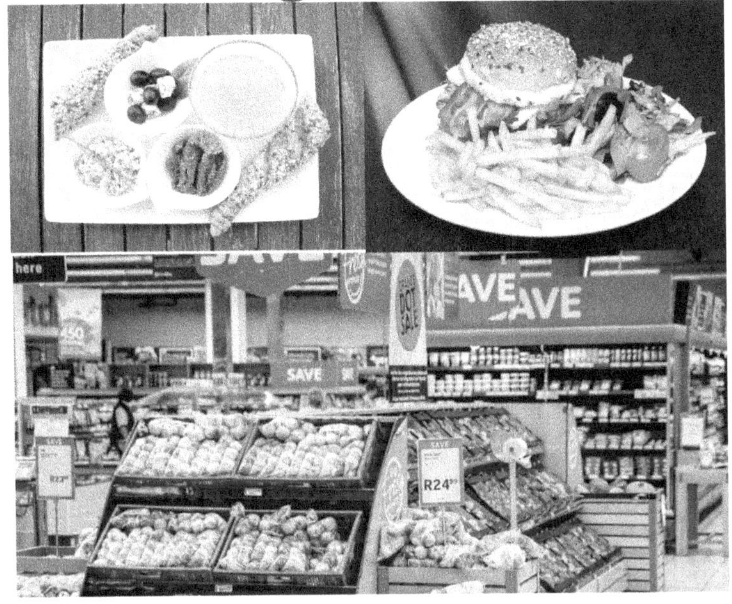

Yet, that doesn't mean you need to think twice about flavor and innovativeness.

Enter the universe of "Rapid and Basic Weeknight Dining experiences," where culinary sorcery occurs instantly.

With these procedures, you can change your weeknight suppers from a rushed undertaking into a wonderful culinary encounter.

Key Dinner Arranging

The key to fast weeknight feasts lies in essential dinner arranging. Pause for a minute every week to frame your meals.

Ponder dishes that require insignificant readiness and cooking time. Consider extras that can be reused into very interesting dinners.

With a dinner plan close by, you'll save time, diminish squander, and limit last-minute takeout choices.

- 30-Minute Wonders:

Who says connoisseur dinners need hours to plan? A plenty of tasty dishes can be prepared shortly or less.

Sautés, pasta dishes, and straightforward protein and vegetable mixes are your closest companions.

One-dish or one-pot recipes are especially effective, as they limit cleanup and cooking steps.

Keep an assortment of these fast recipes close by, and you won't ever be confused for a quick weeknight supper.

- Prep-Ahead Fixings:

Preparing fixings ahead of time is your unmistakable advantage for speedy weeknight feasts.

Invest some energy toward the end of the week washing, slashing, and dividing vegetables and proteins.

These pre-arranged fixings can be put away in the cooler or cooler, fit to be integrated into your weeknight feasts. This recovers time as well as lessens food squander.

- Brighten up Your Storeroom:

A very much supplied storage room is a weeknight fighter's partner. Keep it loaded up with flavors, spices, sauces, and canned merchandise that can change conventional fixings into remarkable dinners.
Sauces like soy sauce, tomato glue, and curry glues can add moment flavor to your dishes. Try different things with various flavors to hoist your weeknight feasts.

- Sheet Container Dinners:

Sheet container dinners are a weeknight wonder. These one-container ponders include throwing your selection of proteins and vegetables with flavors, spreading them out on a baking sheet, and simmering until flawlessness.

The outcome is a tasty, hands-off feast with negligible cleanup. You can make endless varieties to keep your weeknight suppers invigorating.

- The Moment Pot Benefit:

The Moment Pot is a unique advantage for weeknight cooking. A multi-useful machine can sauté, pressure cook, slow cook, and that's only the tip of the iceberg.

With a Moment Pot, you can get ready dishes that normally require long periods of cooking in a small part of the time.

From bean stew to stews and risottos, this kitchen device is a weeknight legend.

- Sound and Fast Other options:

Quick weeknight feasts don't need to be undesirable. Consider integrating lean proteins, entire grains, and a lot of vegetables into your feasts.

Lean protein sources like chicken, turkey, and fish cook rapidly and give fundamental supplements.

Entire grains, for example, quinoa and brown rice can be ready ahead of time or cooked rapidly.

Make vegetables the superstar by involving them as a base or in generous plates of mixed greens.

- Feasting in Style:

Indeed, even on a bustling weeknight, it is feasible to feast in style. A perfectly set table can raise your feast from normal to remarkable.

Utilize appealing dinnerware, set out new blossoms or candles, and make a comfortable air with music.

Feasting in a wonderful climate can transform a hurried supper into a magnificent encounter.

- Weeknight Devours the Go:

Life can be erratic, and some of the time weeknights require feasts in a hurry. Settle on speedy and sound takeout choices from eateries that proposition adjusted, nutritious decisions.

On the other hand, gather a Do-It-Yourself feast with fixings from a neighborhood self-service counter or arranged food segment.

Conclusion:

- Easy Weeknight Enjoyments:

"Quick and Straightforward Weeknight Galas" demonstrate that weeknight meals can be both effective and extraordinary. With just the right amount of key preparation, some kitchen easy routes, and a smidgen of imagination, you can change your weeknight feasts into magnificent culinary encounters.

Whether you're cooking in a short time, utilizing the Moment Pot, or making sheet dish dinners, these techniques offer you a speedy course to tasty weeknight eating.

Express farewell to everyday weeknight suppers and welcome the delight of fast, basic, and delectable dining experiences.

2. 30-Minute Dinners for Occupied Days:

At the point when a bustling weeknight plan holds you back from feeling like you can have a good feast on the table, go after these 10 Speedy Solid Supper Thoughts.

With having 30-minute feasts readily available, you'll have the option to prepare a sound and delightful supper regardless of what your timetable tosses at you.

These Solid Supper Thoughts Are Flavorful And Family-Accommodating.
Before you request takeout or reach for another not exactly solid supper choice or even request everybody to "battle for themselves," we believe you should realize you have choices!

We've gathered together 10 sound supper thoughts that are not difficult to make at home, family-accommodating, and guarantee that you're all ready to plunk down and invest energy with your friends and family while partaking in a nutritious dinner - any evening of the week.

To make it significantly more possible, we've likewise picked 30 minute dinners that incorporate prep-ahead tips that should try and be possible daily or two ahead of time. We want to believe that you find this rundown of supper thoughts accommodating and move you to get cooking!

- The Advantages Of Cooking At Home And Having Supper As A Family

Preparing more feasts at home is one of the very best lifestyle choices and a solid way of life. As per an investigation of in excess of 9,000 individuals distributed in General Wellbeing Nourishment preparing feasts at home was related with weight reduction, eating less calories and fat, and eating more nutritious food sources.

Furthermore, however wellbeing is one of the main reasons we intend to assist individuals with appreciating more home-prepared feasts, we know it's only one of the many advantages of getting into the kitchen.

At the point when a bustling weeknight plan holds you back from feeling like you can have a quality feast on the table, go after these Speedy Solid Supper Thoughts.

With having 30-minute feasts readily available, you'll have the option to prepare a sound and delightful supper regardless of what your timetable tosses at you.

- These Sound Supper Thoughts Are Tasty And Family-Accommodating.

Before you request takeout or reach for another not exactly sound supper choice or even request everybody to "fight for themselves," we maintain that you should realize you have choices!

We've gathered together sound supper thoughts that are not difficult to make at home, family-accommodating, and guarantee that you're all ready to plunk down and invest energy with your friends and family while partaking in a nutritious dinner - any evening of the week.

To make it much more feasible, we've likewise picked 30 minute dinners that incorporate prep-ahead tips that should try and be possible daily or two ahead of time. We truly want to believe that you find this rundown of supper thoughts accommodating and rouse you to get cooking!

- The 5 Insider facts to Feeling Better Quick:
- As A Family:

Preparing more dinners at home is one of the very best lifestyle choices and a sound way of life.

As per an investigation of in excess of 9,000 individuals distributed in General Wellbeing Sustenance preparing feasts at home was related with weight reduction, eating less calories and fat, and eating more nutritious food varieties.

Also, however well being is one of the main reasons we plan to assist individuals with appreciating more home-prepared feasts, we know it's only one of the many advantages of getting into the kitchen.

Research shows that individuals who cook at home versus the people who eat for the most part take-out or café dinners

Take in a normal of 13 pounds less sugar each year
Eat 4 pounds less fat each year

Have essentially highest scores on the Good dieting File

Eat from a more extensive assortment of nutritional categories, acquiring supplements

- Eat more modest parts:

Spend up to 80% less on the expense of every feast

Have better, more joyful, and more intelligent children

Have better family connections

- Simple Egg Roll In A Bowl:

Love egg rolls? This Simple Egg Roll in a Bowl recipe integrates every one of the flavors from scrumptious egg rolls into a one-dish

dinner that is prepared in under 30 minutes and is crammed with veggies! Searching for a healthfully adjusted, without gluten, or Entire 30 Egg Roll in a Bowl recipe? This is all there is to it!

- One-Dish Chicken Fajita Prepare:

Feeling enticed to feast out for supper? Partake in all the sizzle and kind of an eatery in the solace of your own home with our One-Dish Chicken Fajita Prepare! With a fixing rundown of chicken, peppers, and onions and a small bunch of flavors, you can't beat this speedy and simple weeknight supper recipe that is prepared in a short time.

- Skillet Prepared Chicken:

Take the family back to the table for this Whole30-accommodating Skillet Prepared Chicken that is certain to please! Made with pineapple, chime peppers, sweet onions, delicate chicken, and a hand crafted sauce (more straightforward than you suspect!) this skillet dinner is loaded with supplements and flavor. Effectively prepared early on for a fast supper thought.

- Zucchini Turkey Meatballs:

Italian Turkey Zucchini Meatballs are stove heated and met up with only a couple of basic fixings. They make for a fast weeknight dinner and are feast prep and cooler well disposed!

Likewise, they're an extraordinary method for getting a charge out of zucchini in an exquisite manner and a pleasant method for slipping more veggies into your eating regimen!

Appreciate them with no guarantees or throw them in your #1 marinara to present with pasta, zucchini noodles, or spaghetti squash.

- Pork Lettuce Wraps:

Get a flavorful dinner on the table in under 30 minutes with these Pork Lettuce Wraps.

They're fast and tasty and made across the board skillet. Cooked ground pork, sautéed mushrooms, onions, and water chestnuts are stewed in a delightful yet straightforward natively constructed sauce and put into a fresh lettuce leaf.

You can likewise serve these 'bowl-style' over cooked rice or cauliflower rice for another solid supper though.

- Quinoa Spinach Turkey Burgers With Goat Cheddar:

These Quinoa Spinach Turkey Burgers with Goat Cheddar aren't your typical burger.

They needn't bother with a lot of garnishes to make them sparkle since they're now so great similarly as they are.

They're far superior on a bed of greens thrown with extra-virgin olive oil and new lemon juice.

With only 10 minutes of planning time and 15 minutes to concoct them, you'll have a spiced up burger night prepared in heavenly time!

3. One-Pot Marvels:

In the quick moving universe of current life, shuffling various pots and skillets can be a culinary test.

Enter the universe of "One-Pot Wonders," where you can make luscious dinners without the requirement for a broad exhibit of cookware.

These dishes are a demonstration of the excellence of straightforwardness, where a solitary pot turns into the stage for an orchestra of flavors.

With one-pot wonders, you'll encounter the wizardry of comfort, without settling on taste.

- Productivity Meets Flavor:

One-pot wonders are a demonstration of the marriage of productivity and flavor. In a solitary vessel, you can consolidate a variety of fixings, from proteins and vegetables to grains and flavors.

The excellence lies in the layers of flavor that create as these fixings stew and merge together, making an agreeable and adjusted dinner.

- Less Cleanup, Greater Pleasure:

One-pot wonders are not just about cooking; they're tied in with working on the whole culinary experience.

With less pots and dishes to clean, you can appreciate your feast without the overwhelming possibility of a broad cleanup.

This effortlessness reaches out past the kitchen and into the delight of shared dinners, where you can zero in on discussion and association.

- Vast Varieties:

The universe of one-pot wonders is a material of vast conceivable outcomes.

From good stews and consoling risottos to lively paellas and flavorful pan-sears, the choices are restricted exclusively by your creative mind.

You can modify these dishes to suit your taste and dietary inclinations, making feasts that are exceptionally yours.

- Moment Pot Benefits:

The Moment Pot, a cutting edge kitchen wonder, has brought the idea of one-pot cooking higher than ever.

This multi-practical machine consolidates the elements of a strain cooker, slow cooker, and that's just the beginning.

With a Moment Pot, you can set one up pot dishes with speed and accuracy, accomplishing results that normally require hours in a small part of the time.

- Adjusted and Nutritious:

One-pot wonders are not just about comfort; they're about nourishment as well. You can make adjusted and healthy feasts by integrating lean proteins, entire grains, and a rainbow of vegetables.

These dishes are flexible, permitting you to embrace a scope of culinary customs and dietary requirements.

- Fast and Consoling:

Weeknight meals ought to be consoling and fast, and one-pot wonders follow through on the two fronts.

Whether you're making a spirit relieving pot of bean stew, a delightful group of pasta, or a fragrant curry, these dishes give the solace of home-prepared feasts without the tedious exertion.

- Cooking for a Group:

One-pot wonders are ideal for engaging, permitting you to set up a tasty blowout for a social occasion without the pressure of dealing with various dishes.

From relaxed social affairs to formal meals, these dishes are sufficiently flexible to suit any event.

Conclusion:

- One Pot, Bountiful Flavors:

"One-Pot Wonders" are a demonstration of the possibility that in effortlessness, there is overflow.

These dishes work on cooking as well as upgrade the eating experience, offering the ideal mix of flavors and accommodation.

Whether you're a culinary fledgling or a carefully prepared gourmet expert, one-pot wonders permit you to make phenomenal dishes without the requirement for a broad exhibit of cookware.

Express farewell to kitchen confusion and embrace the wizardry of one-pot cooking, where a solitary pot holds the way to culinary pleasure**Chapter 5:**

1. Good dieting Made Scrumptious:

Great Counting calories Made Heavenly: Relishing the Specialty of Nutritious Pleasure

Good dieting Made Scrumptious:

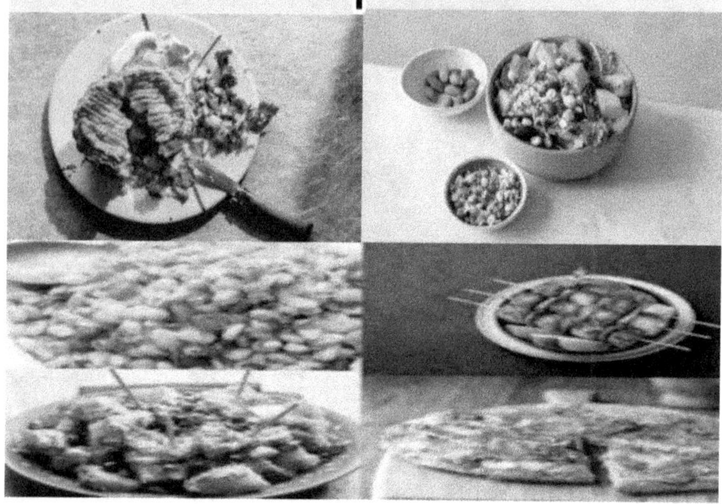

Eating fewer carbs frequently summons pictures of boring dinners, dull servings of mixed greens, and the interminable torture of denying your taste buds.

In any case, imagine a scenario where I let you know that you could partake in the delights of good counting calories while enjoying tasty, healthy feasts. In the realm of

"Good Slimming down Made Heavenly," you set out on a magnificent excursion that demonstrates that eating for wellbeing and delight can coincide agreeably.

- The Force of Flavor Combination:

Great eating fewer carbs doesn't mean you need to forfeit flavor. As a matter of fact, it's a chance to investigate the universe of taste in thrilling and creative ways.

Flavor combination is at the core of good eating less junk food made tasty. It's the craft of joining new fixings, spices, flavors, and flavors to make dishes that entice your sense of taste.

Consider strong curries, lively salsas, and appetizing pan-sears that change ordinary fixings into culinary experiences.

- Healthy and Supplement Rich Fixings:

The groundwork of good counting calories is the choice of healthy and supplement rich fixings.

Organic products, vegetables, lean proteins, entire grains, and vegetables become your partners on this culinary excursion.

With an emphasis on new and natural food varieties, you support your body as well as open the way to excellent taste.

- Cooking Procedures for Most extreme Character:

Counting calories made tasty includes dominating cooking methods that upgrade the kind of your dishes.

Strategies like cooking, barbecuing, and sautéing draw out the regular pleasantness and profundity of fixings.

Preparing with spices and flavors can raise your feasts higher than ever, making an ensemble of taste that leaves your taste buds hitting the dance floor with satisfaction.

- Careful Eating: Appreciate Each Nibble.

Careful eating is an essential part of good counting calories. It's tied in with dialing back, enjoying each nibble, and valuing the surfaces and kinds of your feast.

This training not just permits you to partake in your food all the more yet additionally assists you with perceiving when you're fulfilled, forestalling gorging.

- Difficult exercise: Macros and Micros:

Eating less calories is about balance, both as far as macronutrients and micronutrients.

Macronutrients like proteins, starches, and solid fats assume a part in fulfilling your yearning and giving energy.

Micronutrients, for example, nutrients and minerals guarantee your body works ideally. Finding some kind of harmony brings about feasts that are nutritious as well as flavorful.

- Recipe Remix: Reevaluating Works of art:

Great slimming down made delectable includes reconsidering exemplary dishes.

Rather than wiping out your #1 solace food sources, you can adjust them to accommodate your dietary objectives. Attempt cauliflower pureed potatoes, zucchini noodles, or dark bean brownies.

Recipe remixes make the way for imagination in the kitchen and proposition a new interpretation of old top picks.

- Culinary Investigation: A Universe of Flavors:

Great counting calories made flavorful is a culinary experience. It's an investigation of flavors from around the world.

Embrace the dynamic and various cooking styles of various societies, each offering special and energizing taste encounters.

From Mediterranean to Asian, Center Eastern to Latin American, the universe of flavors is readily available.

- Handcrafted Goodness:

One of the delights of good slimming down made flavorful is the joy of natively constructed feasts.

At the point when you set up your dishes, you have full command over the fixings, bits, and arrangement strategies. You can guarantee that each nibble is a work of art of flavor and sustenance.

Conclusion:

- Appreciate the Excursion:

"Great Eating fewer carbs Made Delectable" is an encouragement to appreciate each part of your dietary process.

It's an investigation of flavors, a festival of new and healthy fixings, and a demonstration of the possibility that great sustenance can be a liberal enjoyment.

The key is to embrace the innovativeness of the kitchen, to investigate a universe of fixings, and to offset flavor with nourishment.

At the point when you approach consuming less calories as a craftsmanship, a wellspring of delight, and a potential chance to enjoy the universe of food, you open the way to great slimming down made flavorful.

It's not just about what's on your plate; it's about the experience of each and every nibble, the delight of culinary investigation, and the amicable association of wellbeing and joy.

2. Supplement Rich Recipes that Satisfy:

Lift Your Wellbeing with Flavor.
In a world loaded up with dietary patterns and superfoods, the mission for adjusted sustenance

can in some cases feel overpowering.

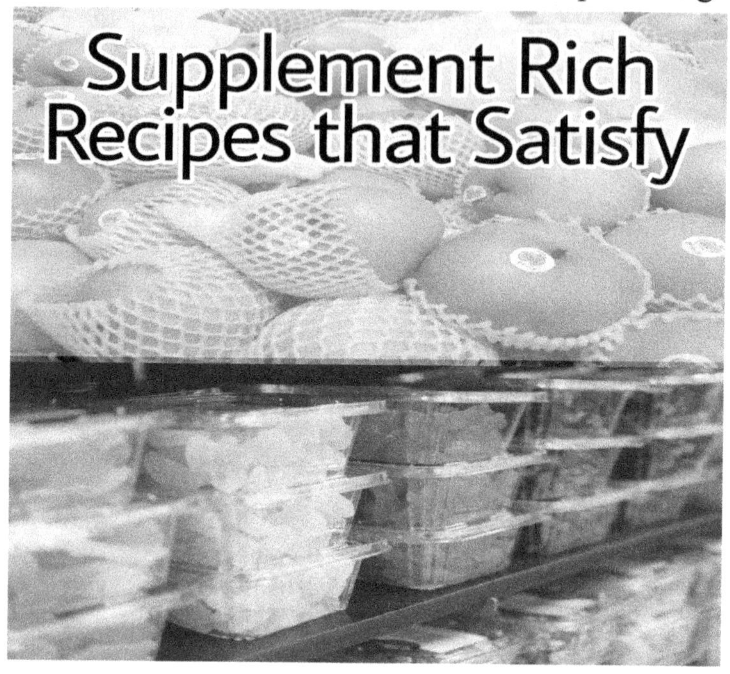

Yet, imagine a scenario where you could upgrade your wellbeing with supplement-rich recipes that satisfy your wholesome requirements as well as entice your taste buds.

Welcome to the domain of "Supplement Rich Recipes that Satisfy," where culinary creativity meets the study of wellbeing.

- The Force of Supplement Thick Fixings:

The center guideline of supplement-rich recipes is outfitting the influence of supplement thick fixings.

These are food sources that sneak up suddenly with regards to nutrients, minerals, cancer prevention agents, and fundamental supplements.

Think salad greens like kale and spinach, superfoods like chia seeds and goji berries, and protein forces to be reckoned with, for example, quinoa and beans. These fixings become the establishment for your culinary manifestations.

- Adjusting Macronutrients for Satiety:

Supplement thickness is only one part of supplement-rich recipes. Adjusting macronutrients - proteins, sugars, and solid fats -

guarantees that your dinners fulfill your appetite while advancing generally prosperity.

A very much organized dish unites lean proteins, complex sugars, and great fats, making a fantastic and refreshing feasting experience.

- Superfood Stars:

Acai, Turmeric, and that's only the tip of the iceberg.
Consolidating superfoods into your recipes is a sign of supplement-rich cooking.

These culinary stars implant your dishes with rich flavors as well as offering plenty of medical advantages. Acai, known for its cell reinforcement properties, can be transformed into energetic dishes.

Turmeric, with its mitigating potential, can add profundity to curries and soups. With superfoods, you're not simply eating; you're feeding your body.

- Fulfilling Enhancements:

Collagen, Omega-3s, and Probiotics.
Supplement-rich recipes go past ordinary fixings. They present enhancements like collagen, omega-3 unsaturated fats, and probiotics into your eating regimen.

Collagen-imbued smoothies improve skin wellbeing, while omega-3-rich salmon advances heart prosperity. Probiotic-rich yogurt bowls are a pleasure for stomach wellbeing.
These enhancements lift your dinners to nourishing forces to be reckoned with.

- Hand crafted Health Elixirs:

Supplement-rich recipes frequently incorporate hand crafted health elixirs. These are drinks intended to support your wellbeing while at the same time enchanting your faculties. Turmeric lattes offer calming goodness. Green smoothies are a wellspring of essentialness. Natural teas like chamomile and ginger alleviate and revive. These elixirs are a day to day custom of health.

- Relishing Zest and Spices:

Tasty Wellbeing Sponsors.
Flavors and spices are a foundation of supplement-rich recipes. They not just add profundity and flavor to your dishes yet additionally bring medical advantages.

Cinnamon can balance out glucose, while ginger can help processing. New spices like basil and mint are plentiful in nutrients and cell reinforcements. These culinary marvels are both heavenly and recuperating.

- Tempting Treats:

Nut Spread Cups, Chia Pudding, from there, the sky's the limit.

Indeed, even liberal treats can be essential for supplement-rich cooking. Nut spread cups can integrate protein and sound fats.

Chia pudding can be injected with fiber and omega-3s. Dull chocolate-shrouded berries can offer cell reinforcements. These wonderful joys guarantee that your health process incorporates snapshots of guilty pleasure.

- Modifying Your Wellbeing Process:

Supplement-rich recipes offer you the adaptability to redo your wellbeing process.

Whether you're trying to help your resistant framework, upgrade your skin, or backing your heart, you can tailor your recipes to satisfy your remarkable health objectives. These recipes become a material for your wellbeing yearnings.

- Determination:

A Culinary Way to Wellbeing

"Supplement Rich Recipes that Satisfy" are a demonstration of the possibility that wellbeing can be a wonderful excursion. It's not necessary to focus on hardship; it's tied in with commending the decency of food.

These recipes are a mix of science and craftsmanship, sustenance and flavor.
At the point when you embrace the universe of supplement-rich cooking, you're not simply eating; you're sustaining your body and soul. You're investigating the kinds of wellbeing and the shades of sustenance.

A culinary way to wellbeing guarantees your feasts are fulfilling as you would prefer buds as well as to your wellbeing yearnings. Thus, let your kitchen become the material where you make supplement-rich recipes that satisfy.

3. Smart Exchanges for Better Cooking:

Lift Your Culinary Abilities.
Cooking isn't just about following recipes; it's a consistently advancing excursion of inventiveness and expertise improvement.

In the realm of "Sagacious Exchanges for Better Cooking," you'll find the specialty of culinary authority through savvy trades and procedures that upgrade your dishes.

These sharp exchanges will enable you to change normal dinners into unprecedented culinary encounters.

- Trade It Out: Shrewd Fixing Replacements:

Canny cooking starts with fixing replacements. Whether you're obliging dietary limitations or essentially searching for a better curve, savvy trades can improve things significantly.

Trade out customary pasta for zucchini noodles or cauliflower rice to eliminate carbs. Supplant weighty cream with a mix of yogurt and milk for a lighter, tart other option.

Try different things with almond flour or coconut flour in baking to make sans gluten treats.

- The Tasty Wizardry of New Spices:

New spices are your distinct advantage for lifting the kind of any dish. Exchanging dried spices for their new partners adds an explosion of energy and smell.

Sprinkle new basil on your custom made pizza, embellish your plate of mixed greens with fragrant cilantro, or use rosemary to mix a meal with hearty goodness. New spices reinvigorate your recipes and proposition a moment redesign in taste.

- Embrace the Umami Extravagance of Mushrooms:

Mushrooms are a sagacious cook's closest companion. These umami-stuffed growths add profundity and intricacy to dishes without the requirement for meat.

Trade out a portion of the ground meat in your stew for slashed mushrooms, making a heartier, more delightful variant.

Portobello mushrooms can be utilized as a substantial burger substitution. By integrating mushrooms, you upgrade flavor as well as lift sustenance.

- Hoist Your Oils and Fats:

Brilliant exchanges reach out to your selection of oils and fats. Trade out customary vegetable oil for better options like olive oil, avocado oil, or coconut oil.

These choices bring a particular flavor as well as proposition a scope of medical advantages. Moreover, think about supplanting margarine with ghee (explained spread) for a nutty, hot extravagance in your cooking.

- Dietary Force to be reckoned with: Cauliflower:

Cauliflower is a flexible, sagacious cook's fantasy. It tends to be changed into a heap of dishes, from cauliflower pounded "potatoes" to cauliflower pizza hull.

This cruciferous vegetable is a low-carb, supplement rich substitute that permits you to partake in your number one solace food varieties while adhering to your dietary objectives.

- Careful Dinner Preparing:

Dinner preparing is the sign of adroit cooking. By devoting a period every week to plan fixings ahead of time, you save time and diminish the pressure of cooking on occupied weeknights.

Hack vegetables, marinate proteins, and piece out grains for simple get together when supper time shows up.

- Redo Your Storage space Staples:

Redesign your storage space staples with superior grade, wellbeing cognizant decisions. Exchange refined white sugar for normal sugars like honey or maple syrup.

Pick entire grains like earthy colored rice, quinoa, and entire wheat pasta over refined choices. Choose low-sodium soy sauce and stocks to control your salt admission.

- Vital Zest Mixes:

Flavors are the core of flavor in your cooking. Sharp cooks comprehend the specialty of creating their flavor mixes.

Explore different avenues regarding hand crafted taco preparing, curry powders, and bean stew zest mixes to make tailor-made flavors that improve your dishes.

- Decreased Sugar Sweets:

Liberal treats don't need to be stacked with sugar. Trade out refined sugar for sugars like stevia, dates, or natural product purees in your baking and sweet recipes. These options add regular pleasantness without the sugar rush and crash.

Conclusion:

The Specialty of Keen Cooking.
"Keen Exchanges for Better Cooking" is a culinary experience that changes your kitchen into an inventive jungle gym.

The craft of shrewd replacements, fixing updates, and capable procedures guarantees that your cooking isn't just about fulfilling your yearning however about charming your sense of taste.

These keen exchanges engage you to make better, more delightful dinners, whether you're obliging dietary inclinations or hoping to upgrade your culinary abilities.

By embracing the craft of sharp cooking, you'll lift your dishes and transform each dinner into a wonderful and careful experience.

Chapter 6:

1. Cooking for Unprecedented Eating Regimens:

Creating Culinary Wizardry with Dietary Accuracy.

Cooking for unprecedented eating regimens isn't about limitation; it's a journey of culinary development and gastronomic enjoyment.

In the domain of "Cooking for Uncommon Eating Regimens," dietary accuracy weds culinary imaginativeness, permitting you to create feasts that stick to explicit dietary necessities as well as tempt your taste buds.

- The Force of Dietary Explicitness:

Remarkable eating regimens incorporate a great many dietary decisions, from veggie lover and vegan ways of life to without gluten, low-carb, and ketogenic slims down.

Every routine accompanies its own arrangement of rules and limitations. The craft of cooking for uncommon eating regimens is to embrace these dietary particulars and make feasts that adjust flawlessly.

- Fixing Replacements with Pizazz:

Cooking for unprecedented eating regimens frequently includes shrewd fixing replacements.

Supplanting regular fixings with inventive options maintains dietary limitations while adding new components of flavor.

Trade out customary pasta with spiralized zucchini or use cauliflower as a flexible base for dishes that are both sans gluten and low in carbs.

- Energetic Plant-Based Manifestations:

Veggie lovers and vegan eating regimens are a material for innovativeness. With an emphasis on plant-based fixings, your culinary investigation brings you into a universe of energetic vegetables, vegetables, and meat choices.

Exchange out creature items for imaginative plant-based proteins like tempeh, seitan, or tofu. Investigate the assorted flavors and surfaces of the plant realm.

- Embracing the Universe of Sans gluten Grains:

Sans gluten counts calories require a hug of a world without wheat, grain, or rye. Be that as it may, this is a long way from an impediment.

The universe without gluten grains is an exquisite experience. Exchange conventional flour for choices like almond flour, coconut flour, or rice flour to make delectable sans gluten heated products.

- Adjusted Low-Carb Miracles:

Low-carb eating regimens are about balance. By decreasing starch consumption and consolidating lean proteins, solid fats, and fiber-rich vegetables, you make dinners that keep you feeling full and empowered.

Trade out high-carb side dishes with cauliflower rice or simmered Brussels sprouts, transforming your plate into a low-carb wonderland.

- Ketogenic Culinary Speculative chemistry:

The ketogenic diet takes low-carb cooking to a higher level. It's tied in with entering a condition of ketosis where the body consumes fat for fuel. Embrace solid fats like avocados, olive oil, and coconut oil to supplant customary carb sources. Exchange dull sides for keto-accommodating choices like mashed cauliflower or zucchini noodles.

- Careful Feast Preparing:

Dietary accuracy frequently includes feast preparing. By committing time to design and set up your dinners ahead of time, you guarantee that your dietary necessities are met consistently.

Cleave, marinate, and segment out your elements for simple get together when supper time shows up. Feast preparing isn't just a life hack yet in addition a careful practice that keeps you on target with your eating routine.

- Tasty Limitations, Vast Innovativeness:

Cooking for uncommon eating regimens shows that dietary limitations need not limit your culinary innovativeness.

By understanding the complexities of various weight control plans and embracing the universe of fixing replacements, you can make dinners that honor your dietary requirements while enjoying an embroidery of flavors.

Conclusion:

Culinary Accuracy and Masterfulness.
"Cooking for Remarkable Eating Regimens" is the exemplification of dietary accuracy mixed with culinary creativity.

About making feasts line up with your dietary decisions, whether you're veggie lover, sans gluten, low-carb, or ketogenic.

These feasts are not just about adherence; they're tied in with enjoying the culinary excursion of culinary imagination, and they demonstrate that exceptional eating regimens can be an entryway to magnificent gastronomy.

2 . Without Gluten, Vegan, and Keto-Obliging Recipes:

A Culinary Orchestra of Dietary Concordance. Exploring dietary inclinations and limitations doesn't mean you need to forfeit flavor and imagination in the kitchen.

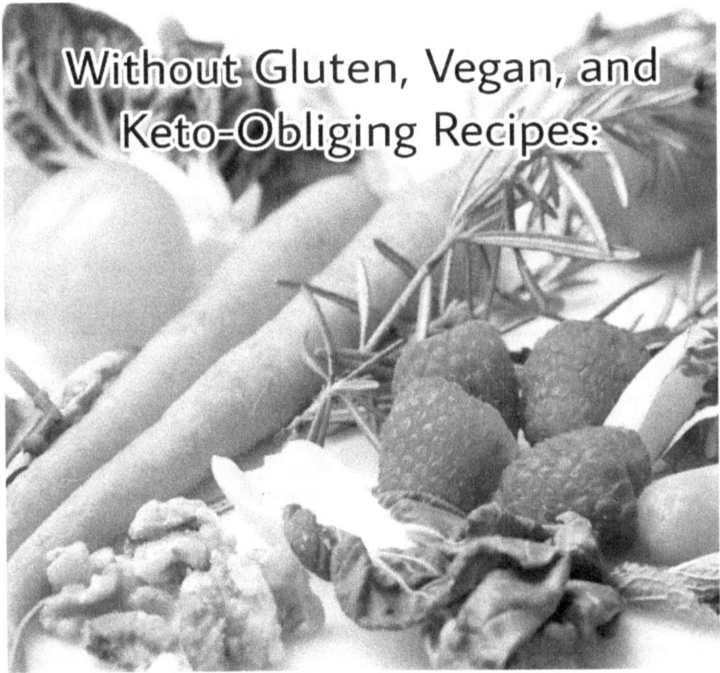

In the realm of "Without Gluten, Vegan, and Keto-Obliging Recipes," you'll leave on a culinary excursion that fits dietary requirements with scrumptious feasts that charm the faculties.

- Dumping Gluten with Fervor:

Sans gluten cooking is a culinary experience. It's tied in with investigating the flavors and surfaces of grains like quinoa, rice, and corn while abandoning customary wheat-based flours.

Trade out wheat pasta for rice or lentil pasta to make without gluten pasta dishes that are similarly fulfilling. Embrace almond flour, coconut flour, or custard flour for baking and find the delight of sans gluten treats.

- Vegan Ponders:

A Plant-Based Orchestra.
Vegan cooking is an orchestra of plant-based ponders. It's tied in with creating dishes that

praise the lively universe of vegetables, vegetables, and meat choices.

Trade out creature proteins with fixings like tempeh, tofu, or chickpeas to make good and protein-rich veggie lover dinners.

Cooked vegetables, dynamic servings of mixed greens, and imaginative grain bowls add profundity to your veggie lover collection.

- Keto Pleasures:

Embracing Solid Fats.
The ketogenic diet is tied in with embracing solid fats while lessening sugars.

Trade out high-carb sides with keto-accommodating options like pounded cauliflower or spiralized zucchini.

Exchange dull backups for avocado and olive oil-based manifestations. The outcome is a menu brimming with keto delights that are both fulfilling and restorative.

- Adjusted Morning meals:

The morning feast establishes the vibe for the afternoon. Trade out customary breakfast oats for sans gluten oats finished off with new berries and a dab of Greek yogurt.

Make good vegan breakfast burritos with mixed tofu and a rainbow of sautéed vegetables.

For those following a keto routine, enjoy avocado and poached eggs, a match made in keto paradise.

- Noon Disclosures:

Lunch is your late morning fuel, and you can create delightful dinners to support you.

Make sans gluten grain plates of mixed greens with a variety of vivid vegetables and your decision of protein. Veggie lover snacks can include good grain bowls with beans and broiled vegetables, sprinkled with an exquisite tahini dressing. For a keto-accommodating choice, enjoy a delectable spinach and feta stuffed chicken bosom.

- Supper Enjoyments for All:

Supper is where culinary inventiveness sparkles. For a sans gluten supper, enjoy spaghetti squash with a delicious tomato and basil sauce.

Vegan meals can incorporate a rich portobello mushroom steak with garlic crushed cauliflower. A keto-accommodating supper could be a rich salmon filet with a side of sautéed asparagus.

- Sweet Treats and Pastries:

Sweets are a guilty pleasure for every dietary inclination. For without gluten fans, almond flour-based brownies and flourless chocolate cake are rich and fulfilling.

Veggie lover treats incorporate smooth coconut rice pudding mixed with sweet-smelling flavors. On the keto front, have a great time with dull chocolate avocado mousse or coconut almond fat bombs.

- A Dietary Orchestra:

"Without Gluten, Vegan, and Keto-Obliging Recipes" is a dietary ensemble that orchestrates flavor, wellbeing, and dietary accuracy.

These recipes demonstrate that you can take care of dietary inclinations and limitations without settling on culinary inventiveness.

Embrace the universe of fixing replacements and creative cooking procedures, and let your kitchen become a sanctuary for dietary concordance.

A culinary excursion raises each feast, from breakfast to supper, and changes treats into sweet enjoyments for all.

Chapter 7:

1. Cooking for a Gathering:

From Kitchen Bedlam to Culinary Achievement. Cooking for a gathering can be an overwhelming undertaking, with the potential for disorder in the kitchen and nervousness over fulfilling different preferences and dietary inclinations.

Be that as it may, it's likewise an open door to exhibit your culinary abilities and unite individuals over a delectable feast.

In the realm of "Cooking for a Gathering," you'll get familiar with the specialty of arranging, readiness, and show that changes a possibly distressing occasion into a culinary victory.

- The Test of Scale:

Cooking for a gathering isn't just about increasing a recipe; it's tied in with adjusting your cooking abilities to serve a large number.

The test lies in guaranteeing that each plate is served hot, new, and delectable, even with a bigger headcount. This requires shrewd preparation and reasonable techniques.

- Culminating the Menu:

Begin by making a menu that adjusts assortment, dietary contemplations, and occasional fixings.

Think about the inclinations and dietary limitations of your visitors, offering choices for veggie lovers, vegetarians, or those with sensitivities. A balanced menu guarantees that everybody at the table feels included.

- Shopping Keenly:

Cooking for a gathering starts at the supermarket. Make an itemized shopping list, taking into account the amounts required for the bigger servings.

Purchase in mass when conceivable to save money on costs and diminish squander. New fixings ought to be top quality, guaranteeing that your dishes sparkle.

- Proficient Prep Work:

The way to outcome in cooking for a gathering is effective prep work. Devote time before the occasion to slash, marinate, and segment out fixings.

This recovers time during the cooking system as well as permits you to partake in the organization of your visitors.

- Dominating Make-Ahead Dishes:

Decide on make-ahead dishes that can be arranged to some degree or completely ahead of time. Lasagnas, galoshes, and marinated servings of mixed greens are wonderful models.

These dishes permit you to zero in on your visitors as opposed to being caught in the kitchen.

- The Wizardry of One-Pot Marvels:

One-pot and one-container recipes are a lifeline while cooking for a gathering.

They limit the quantity of pots and containers being used, diminishing both cooking time and cleanup. Dishes like paella, jambalaya, or sautés give a tasty, generous feast without the kitchen bedlam.

- Buffet-Style Administration:

Buffet-style administration is a well disposed way to deal with serving a gathering.

Visitors can pick the bits and mixes that suit their inclinations, and you can keep a coordinated stream in the kitchen. Set up a lovely show with different dishes, and permit your visitors to serve themselves.

- Timing Is Everything:

Guaranteeing that each dish is fit to be served simultaneously requires exact timing.

Use clocks and have an efficient timetable for cooking, warming, and plating. A warm broiler or scraping dishes can assist with keeping food at the right temperature until now is the ideal time to eat.

- Trimmings and Show:

The specialty of embellishing and show lifts your dishes from standard to uncommon. New spices, eatable blossoms, and bright sauces add a visual allure that supplements the flavors. Get some margin to embellish your dishes, and your visitors will be in for a brilliant treat.

- Culinary Victory and Happiness:

"Cooking for a Gathering" isn't just about taking care of individuals; it's tied in with making an essential culinary encounter.

With cautious preparation, productive planning, and brilliant methodologies, you can transform a possibly turbulent occasion into a culinary victory.

You'll fulfill the cravings of your visitors as well as make a warm and welcoming climate that cultivates association and euphoria.

In this way, embrace the test, cook with adoration, and transform your social events into culinary festivals.

2. Working with and Connecting Without any problem:

The Specialty of Consistent Communication.
Working with and connecting effectively is an expertise that changes each communication into a liquid and useful trade.

Whether you're driving a gathering, showing a class, or simply captivating in a cordial discussion, excelling at easy help and commitment makes the cycle smoother and more significant.

- Clear Openness is Of the utmost importance:

The underpinning of working with and connecting effectively is clear correspondence.

Express your thoughts, questions, and assumptions succinctly and straightforwardly. The more straightforward your correspondence, the smoother the association.

Utilize basic and clear language, staying away from language or tangled clarifications.

- Undivided attention: A Scaffold to Commitment.

Undivided attention is the scaffold that interfaces you to your crowd. It's tied in with focusing entirely on the speaker, posing significant inquiries, and giving criticism that shows you figure out their viewpoint.

At the point when individuals feel appreciated and esteemed, they're bound to draw in with excitement.

- Open and Comprehensive Climate:

Establish an open and comprehensive climate where everybody feels happy with sharing their considerations and thoughts.

Empower cooperation and be available to different viewpoints. Encourage an air of trust and regard, where individuals have a good sense of reassurance communicating their thoughts.

- Very much Organized Connection:

Very much organized corporations make help and commitment a breeze. Have an unmistakable plan or plan for your collaboration, whether it's a gathering, a class, or a relaxed discussion. Keep conversations on target, and give clear courses.

This construction assists members with knowing what's in store and how to really contribute.

- Enabling Others:

Engaging others to start to lead the pack can be a strong help instrument. Urge members to share their experiences and take on dynamic jobs in the collaboration.

This conveys the responsibility as well as enables people to take responsibility for conversation.

- Visual Guides and Intelligent Devices'

Integrate visual guides and intuitive instruments to upgrade commitment. Visual components, like outlines, charts, and slides, can explain complex ideas.

Intuitive apparatuses like surveys or meetings to generate new ideas welcome cooperation and make the association seriously captivating.

- Utilization of Innovation:

Influence innovation to work with and connect effectively, particularly in virtual communications.

Video conferencing, visit stages, and online joint effort instruments can smooth out correspondence and make it more available. Embrace innovation that upgrades instead of prevents commitment.

- Careful Using time productively:

Compelling using time effectively is indispensable for consistent assistance and commitment.

Regard members' time by beginning and finishing the cooperation as booked.

Distribute time for central issues, conversations, and back and forth discussions to keep the association on target.

- Adjusting Talking and Tuning in:

Working with and drawing in are a two-way road. While you might be driving the collaboration, guarantee a harmony among talking and tuning in. Take into account stops to allow others to answer and contribute.

This unique keeps all interested parties and makes for a really captivating encounter.

- Look for Nonstop Improvement:

Continuously look for ways of upgrading your help and commitment abilities.

Request criticism from members to comprehend what functioned admirably and what could be gotten to the next level.
Adjust your methodology in light of illustrations gained from every connection.

Conclusion:

- The Specialty of Easy Cooperation:

Working with and connecting effectively is the specialty of making a consistent and significant trade with others.

It's about clear correspondence, undivided attention, and encouraging a comprehensive climate.

With very much organized collaborations, innovation, and careful using time effectively, you can make each connection a breeze.

Recall that the way to dominate this craftsmanship lies in consistent improvement and a promise to make each cooperation seriously captivating, canny, and pleasant for all included.

Chapter 8:

1. Overall Flavors, Neighborhood Trimmings:

A Culinary Experience in Your Kitchen.

In the present globalized world, the culinary scene has changed into an energetic embroidery of overall flavors, displaying the different fixings, recipes, and customs of endless societies.

At the core of this scrumptious excursion lies a lovely idea: "Overall Flavors, Neighborhood Trimmings." This expression epitomizes the possibility that you can investigate worldwide foods and enjoy outlandish dishes utilizing locally accessible fixings, squarely in your own kitchen.

- Worldwide Motivation, Nearby Fixings:

Overall flavors are an encouragement to venture to the far corners of the planet through your taste buds.

Whether you're longing for the intriguing flavors of India, the ameliorating pasta dishes of Italy, or the searing kinds of Mexico, the world's culinary legacy is readily available.

It's really thrilling that you can make these dishes with neighborhood trimmings, making global food open and advantageous.

- Worldwide Storage room Staples;

Building a worldwide storage room is the most vital phase in your culinary experience.

Stock up on flexible fixings like olive oil, garlic, onions, and different flavors that structure the groundwork of numerous cooking styles.

Soy sauce, rice vinegar, and miso glue are key components in Asian cooking, while canned tomatoes and dried pasta are fundamental for Italian dishes.

A worldwide storeroom guarantees you have the nuts and bolts to investigate overall flavors.

- Ranchers' Business sectors and Neighborhood Makers:

Neighborhood trimmings can frequently be tracked down solidly locally. Visit ranchers' business sectors and nearby makers to find new, occasional fixings that line up with the culinary practices of your picked food.

From ranch new produce to distinctive cheeses and meats, you'll be astounded at the wealth of privately obtained fixings that can move your taste buds all over the planet.

- Finding Ethnic Supermarkets:

Ethnic supermarkets are covered up treasures for investigating overall flavors.

These business sectors convey novel fixings well defined for different foods, permitting you to reproduce worldwide dishes legitimately.

Whether it's Mexican business sectors with dried chiles and masa harina, or Center Eastern business sectors loaded with outlandish flavors and safeguarded lemons, these shops open up a universe of culinary conceivable outcomes.

- Adjusting Recipes Inventively:

Adjusting recipes inventively is a sign of overall flavors with neighborhood trimmings.

Feel free to make fixing replacements in view of what's accessible locally. On the off chance that a recipe requires a particular kind of fish that is not promptly tracked down in your space, search out a privately obtained, reasonable other option.

Newness and quality frequently outweigh severe adherence to the recipe.

- Neighborhood Combination Enjoyments.

Embrace the possibility of combining food with a neighborhood contort. Mix the kinds of global dishes with neighborhood trimmings to make imaginative, heavenly outcomes.

For instance, imbue your custom made pizza with the smoky substance of a nearby grill sauce or plan sushi rolls including territorial fish.

- Local area and Culinary Association:

Overall flavors with neighborhood trimmings offer a novel chance to interface with your local area and back nearby makers.

By obtaining fixings locally, you partake in the freshest produce as well as add to the maintainability of nearby farming and economy.

- Worldwide Experience from Your Kitchen:

"Overall Flavors, Neighborhood Trimmings" changes your kitchen into a worldwide experience.

It's tied in with investigating assorted societies and cooking styles through your culinary manifestations.

With the world as your motivation and nearby fixings as your material, you can set out on a gastronomic excursion that commends the kinds of the world while regarding the produce and customs of your area.

It's a heavenly mix of worldwide culture and neighborhood local area that unites individuals through the all inclusive language of food.

2. Examining Overall Food sources in Your Kitchen:

A Culinary Endeavor.

In this present reality where global travel isn't generally a choice, your kitchen turns into the doorway to investigating the world's assorted and enticing cooking styles.

"Researching Overall Food sources in Your Kitchen" is an excursion of culinary revelation that rises above borders, all from the solace of your home.

In this way, secure your cover, snatch your visa (or recipe book), and we should leave on an exhilarating endeavor into the worldwide gastronomy scene.

- Culinary Topography:

Envision your kitchen as a guide, with different districts of the world ready to be investigated.

Every region offers unmistakable flavors, fixings, and cooking procedures.

Begin by choosing a nation or locale that interests you, and dive into its culinary culture. Whether it's the striking and hot dishes of Thailand, the good and exquisite passage of France, or the encouraging and sweet-smelling manifestations of India, anything is possible for you.

- The Worldwide Storage room:

Building a worldwide storage room is the underpinning of your endeavor. Stock your racks with fundamental fixings that length different cooking styles.

Olive oil, garlic, onions, and a determination of spices and flavors like cumin, coriander, and paprika are flexible staples.

Soy sauce, coconut milk, curry glue, and fish sauce are fundamental for Asian dishes, while staples like canned tomatoes, pasta, and Parmesan cheddar are key parts of Italian cooking.

- Nearby Fixings, Worldwide Flavors:

One of the delights of researching overall food varieties is finding that numerous worldwide dishes can be arranged utilizing privately obtained fixings.

Search out adjacent ranchers' business sectors and neighborhood makers to track down new, occasional produce and distinctive merchandise that line up with global culinary practices.

Privately developed vegetables, meats, and cheeses frequently work wonderfully in recipes from around the world.

- Culinary Investigations in Ethnic Business sectors:

Daring to ethnic supermarkets opens up a gold mine of bona fide fixings. These business sectors offer a large number of items interesting to different foods.

You can find everything from interesting flavors and extraordinary natural products to specialty sauces and grains.

Investigate the walkways and extend your culinary skylines with fixings that transport your kitchen to various pieces of the globe.

- Innovative Transformations:

While examining overall food varieties, don't hesitate for even a moment to get innovative. Adjusting recipes with accessible nearby fixings is important for the experience.

Assuming a recipe requires a fixing that is difficult to find in your space, contemplate what nearby options you can utilize.

The key is to keep up with the embodiment of the dish while embracing the flavors and produce accessible in your district.

- Combination Cooking at Home:

Combination cooking is one more thrilling part of your culinary excursion. It's tied in with mixing the kinds of various world foods in imaginative and creative ways.

For example, why not wed the smoky substance of a neighborhood grill sauce with Mexican cooking to make a novel and flavorful combination?

The potential outcomes are inestimable when you're the gourmet expert of your worldwide kitchen.

- Local area Association through Food:

Examining overall food varieties in your kitchen additionally brings your local area closer.

At the point when you purchase from neighborhood ranchers and makers, you support the manageability of nearby horticulture and add to the development of your local area's culinary culture. Imparting your worldwide culinary manifestations to loved ones can prompt a rich trade of flavors and encounters.

- Culinary Discretion from Home:

"Exploring Overall Food Sources in Your Kitchen" is a type of culinary tact. It's tied in with separating social hindrances and encouraging an appreciation for the flavors and customs of the world.

By investigating worldwide cooking in your kitchen, you become a worldwide representative, sharing the sorcery of food as a widespread language.

This culinary undertaking praises the world's culinary variety while manufacturing associations between individuals, societies, and networks. An experience sustains both body and soul, and everything unfurls solidly in your own special kitchen.

Chapter 9:

1. Baking and Treats:

A Heavenly Excursion into the Sweet Side of Life.
The specialty of baking is something other than blending fixings; it's a supernatural change of straightforward components into delicious enjoyments that summon sentimentality and

solace.

Baking and Treats

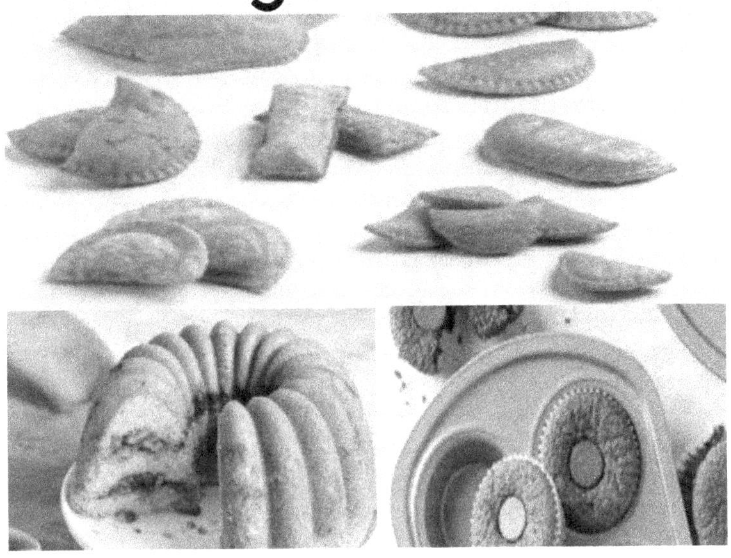

Whether you're preparing treats, cakes, or cakes, "Baking and Treats" is an investigation of the sweet side of life, where the smell of new heated products fills your kitchen and the delight of guilty pleasure makes you feel good inside.

- The Sweet-smelling Speculative chemistry of Baking:

The second you step into a kitchen where baking is in progress, you're welcomed by an orchestra of fragrances.

The warm, rich aroma of chocolate chip treats, the encouraging smell of a vanilla cake, and the fiery scent of cinnamon rolls are commitments of delectability to come.

Baking is a fragrant speculative chemistry that changes fixings into tangible joys.

- The Solace of Custom:

Baking holds an extraordinary spot in our souls since it's frequently attached to custom.

Grandmother's popular fruity dessert, Father's mysterious brownie recipe, or Mother's natively constructed bread - these treats convey the kinds of affection and sentimentality. Baking unites ages and makes enduring recollections.

- The Study of Pleasantness:

Baking is both a workmanship and a science. It includes exact estimations, temperature control, and amazing luck.

From the science of raising specialists to the complexities of flavor matching, each sweet treat is the consequence of a fragile harmony between fixings and methods.

- Imaginative Material:

Baking is an imaginative material where you can put yourself out there. Whether you're enhancing a cake with unpredictable plans, exploring different avenues regarding interesting flavor mixes, or giving exemplary recipes on your own, every creation is an impression of your creative mind and enthusiasm.

- A General Language of Euphoria:

Baking rises above lines and dialects. The delight that comes from gnawing into a newly heated croissant in a comfortable Parisian bistro is a similar bliss as enjoying a warm cup of banana bread in an unassuming community pastry shop.

Baking is an all inclusive language of euphoria that interfaces individuals across the globe.

- Baking as Taking care of oneself:

Baking isn't just about satisfying others; it's likewise a type of taking care of oneself.
There's a helpful thing about
playing batter, estimating fixings, and making wonderful baked goods. Baking permits you to de-stress and articulate your thoughts, all while indulging yourself with the rewards for so much hard work.

- Sweet Treat for Friends and family:

Baking is a demonstration of adoration. Whether it's surprising a companion with a clump of natively constructed treats or baking a cake for a friend or family member's birthday, the demonstration of baking for others shows you give it a second thought. It's a wonderful method for lighting up somebody's day.

- Baking as a Practice:

Baking practices mark extraordinary events and occasions. From gingerbread houses at Christmas to hot cross buns at Easter, these heated products convey the heaviness of custom and become emblematic of the time.

Baking customs assist with making a feeling of congruity and association with the past.

- Extravagance and Festivity:

At long last, baking is about guilty pleasure and festivity. It's tied in with enjoying the sweet minutes throughout everyday life and celebrating in the easily overlooked details.

A warm biscuit with your morning espresso, a birthday cake imparted to companions, or a newly heated pie on a languid Sunday - these are snapshots of festivity and unadulterated, pure delight.

"Baking and Treats" is an excursion into the sweet side of life, where each recipe is a wonderful source of both pain and joy, each smell is a commitment of joy, and each nibble is a festival of the straightforward delights.

It's a universe of innovativeness, custom, and association that fills your kitchen with warmth and your heart with satisfaction.

Whether you're an accomplished dough puncher or simply starting to investigate the universe of treats, each experience into the universe of baking is a heavenly one.

So preheat that broiler, wear your cover, and let the baking start!

2. Satisfy Your Sweet Tooth the Insightful Way:

Fulfilling Desires with Tasty Well Being Cognizant Decisions.
Fulfilling your sweet tooth doesn't need to mean giving up to sweet extravagances that leave you with responsibility and sugar crashes.

The insightful method for satisfying your sweet desires is to pursue careful decisions that consolidate the happiness of desserts with the insight of wellbeing and cognizant living.

How about we investigate how you can please your taste buds while remembering your prosperity.

- Embrace Nature's Sweets:

Nature gives an abundance of sweet choices that can fulfill your desires without the disadvantages of refined sugar.

Organic products like berries, apples, and oranges offer normal pleasantness alongside nutrients, fiber, and cell reinforcements.

Make lively natural product servings of mixed greens, mix up smoothies, or basically appreciate new organic products as a magnificent sweet.

- Savvy Baking Trades:

With regards to baking, you can make sagacious trades to diminish sugar without compromising flavor. Supplant refined sugar with regular sugars like honey, maple syrup, or dates in your recipes.

These choices add a rich pleasantness that matches magnificently with different heated merchandise, from treats to biscuits.

- Nut Margarine Nirvana:

Nut margarines, like almond, cashew, or peanut butter, are your pass to sweet guilty pleasure with added sustenance.

Spread them on entire grain toast, sprinkle them over cereal, or plunge apple cuts for a smooth, protein-stuffed treat.

Nut margarines convey a wonderful equilibrium between pleasantness and solid fats.

- Yogurt Parfait Flawlessness:

Yogurt parfaits are a canny method for getting a charge out of pleasantness while supporting your probiotic consumption.

Layer Greek yogurt with a new natural product, a shower of honey, and a sprinkle of granola for a delicious and nutritious sweet.
The smooth surface and regular pleasantness make it an inside and out.

- Dull Chocolate Pleasures:

Dull chocolate is the modern decision for those with a sweet tooth. It's lower in sugar than milk chocolate and flaunts heart-sound cell reinforcements.

A square or two of top notch dim chocolate can extinguish your desires and give a portion of extravagance without the sugar rush.

- Frozen Natural product Pops:

Make your frozen natural product drops by mixing ready natural products like mangoes, strawberries, or peaches and freezing them in popsicle molds. These natively constructed treats offer the nostalgic joy of a popsicle while being liberated from counterfeit sugars and additives.

- Heat with Entire Grains:

Entire grains like oats, entire wheat flour, and quinoa flour are phenomenal augmentations to your prepared merchandise.

They grant a nutty pleasantness and a large group of nourishing advantages. Have a go at baking treats, biscuits, and cakes with entire grains for a wellbeing cognizant and sweet experience.

- Careful Part Control:

Satisfying your sweet tooth smart style likewise includes careful piece control. As opposed to enjoying a goliath cut of cake, relish a more modest piece.

Take as much time as necessary to partake in each chomp, and you'll find that a tiny amount makes a huge difference when you're aware of each and every significant piece.

- Specialty of Zest Mixing:

Flavors like cinnamon, nutmeg, and cardamom add profundity and warmth to your sweet manifestations. These fragrant flavors raise your treats with a brilliant flavor help while limiting the requirement for inordinate sugar.

- Equilibrium and Assortment:

Equilibrium and assortment are critical to satisfying your sweet tooth the adroit way. It's tied in with integrating a different scope of desserts into your eating regimen, from new organic products to prepared merchandise, and enjoying balance.

By embracing a balanced methodology, you can partake in the joys of pleasantness while keeping a wellbeing cognizant way of life.

Conclusion:

Sweet Fulfillment with Sagacious Decisions.
"Satisfy Your Sweet Tooth the Sagacious Way"
is tied in with embracing a heavenly, wellbeing
cognizant way to deal with fulfilling your sweet
desires.

Nature's abundance, careful trades, and the
innovative utilization of entire fixings change
your treats into savvy decisions that take care of
both your taste buds and prosperity.

This wise methodology empowers you to enjoy
pleasantness without settling for less, leaving
you with a fulfilled sweet tooth and a feeling of
prosperity.

In this way, feel free to take pleasure in the
realm of pleasantness with your recently
discovered sharp insight

3. Baking Tips and Misdirects:

Baking Tips and Misdirects The Specialty of Making Compelling Sweets Baking is a magnificent blend of artificer and wisdom, where a hint of inventiveness and a spot of delicacy meetup to make sweets that warm the heart and allure the taste kids.

" Baking Tips and Bamboozles" is your mysterious form for outstripping at baking. How about we jump into the macrocosm of ranges, blenders, and spatulas, and reveal the numbers and procedures that will raise your heated wares to an advanced position.

Begin with Quality Fixings' The underpinning of any outstanding hotted great falsehoods in the nature of the seasoning. select new eggs, great flour, and unalloyed concentrates.

Premium seasoning can have a recognizable effect on the taste and face of your last creation.

Room Temperature is Critical previous to plunging into your baking experience, guarantee that seasoning like eggs, margarine, and dairy particulars are at room temperature.

This step guarantees in any event, blending and better fuse of seasoning in your player. Measure with delicacy Baking is a wisdom, and exact estimations are abecedarian.

Put coffers into a reliable kitchen scale and estimate mugs and ladles to guarantee you get the specific estimates for your fashions.

A little step can yield critical advancements in your set products.

The witchery of Filtering Filtering your dry seasoning, analogous to flour, cocoa, and incinerating greasepaint, could appear to be a minor detail, still it's an unmistakable advantage in baking.

Filtering eliminates protrusions and circulates air through the dry seasoning, egging lighter and airy issues.

Dominating the Creaming Strategy The creaming strategy is the riddle behind delicate and glacial galettes and treats.

Beat together margarine and sugar until the combination is light and featherlight. This cycle consolidates air, which brings about a sensitive morsel structure in your heated products.

Temperature Control Watch out for your cookstove's temperature.
A cook stove thermometer can help you with guaranteeing your toaster is acclimated precisely.

Baking at the right temperature is vital for incinerating and amazing issues. use a Stove Thermometer Cookstove temperatures can be surprisingly incorrect.

A cookstove thermometer is a little yet abecedarian device to guarantee your toaster is at the right temperature.

This straightforward step can save your sensitive baked goods from transubstantiation into culinary disasters.

Cool Down Step by step When your baking magnum number is out of the cookstove, oppose the coercion to dive in right down.

Allow it to cool in the prospect a many moments previous to moving it to a line rack. Chilling off sluggishly guarantees indeed face and flavors.

The Force of Material Paper Material paper is a dough puncher's dearest companion.

It forestalls staying and guarantees simple expatriation of your instantiations from the dish.

A straightforward trick makes the remittal a breath. Do not Overmix Overmixing can be the defeat of your heated wares.

It can prompt extreme galettes and leathery treats. Mix just until the seasonings are joined to negotiate the ideal face.

Embrace the Rest Time frame A many fusions and blockbuster profit from a rest period in the fridge.

Resting permits the seasoning to combine and brings about better face and flavor.

Try not to rush the cycle; give your admixture or megahit time to chill.

Enhancing Artfulness With respects to enhancing, put coffers into quality canalizing tips and exercise your capacities.

A faultlessly stretched cutlet or treat aesthetics drinking as well as adds a fresh subcaste of pleasure. continuity with incentive Working with incentive can be scary, yet continuity is the key.

Allow the batter to rise meetly, and your chuck will compensate you with an inconceivable face and flavor.

" Baking Tips and Beguiles" is your pass to incinerating achievement.

These numbers and strategies can change your heated wares into compelling sweets that have an enduring effect.

Whether you are a precisely prepared dough puncher or simply beginning your excursion in the realm of flour and sugar, these clever tips and

Hoodwinks will help you with outstripping at baking and make great treats that give pleasure to your kitchen and those fortunate enough to taste your instantiations.

Chapter 10:

1. Kitchen Hacks:

Kitchen Hacks and Tips Your Backup course of action to Culinary Strength.

The kitchen is where culinary charm happens, still it can moreover be a place of maturation and confusion.

Kitchen Hacks

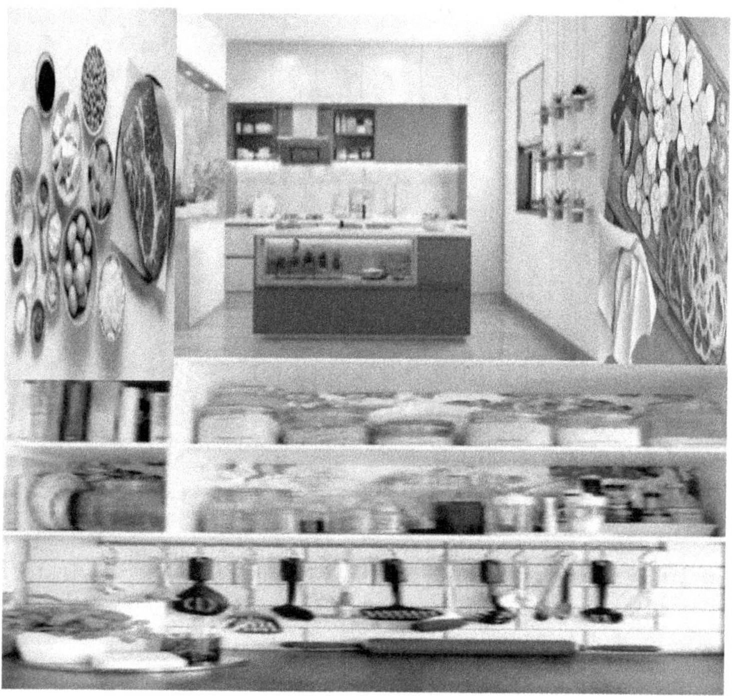

Enter the universe of" Kitchen Hacks and Tips," where culinary erudition meets sly simple courses to change your time in the kitchen from an everyday task to a culinary encounter.

We ought to test these sharp hoodwinks that will make your getting ready and amuse arranging further viable and pleasant.

The significant Onion stunt Onions are a kitchen boss, still they can convey slashes to your eyes, both straightforwardly and from a genuine perspective.

To delay from crying while simultaneously slicing onions, paper this hack cool the onion in the cooler for two or three minutes past to cutting.

Cold onions release less eye-compounding combinations, keeping you dry-checked out and ready to cook.

Basic Garlic Stripping garlic can be a long errand. To make it a breath, self-destruct the garlic bulb, place the cloves in a glass vessel, and shake predominantly.

The skin will loosen, simplifying it to separate and strip the cloves.

Mature Avocados fleetly No really believing that your avocados will advance commonly.

To speed up the cycle, place an immature avocado in a paper sack with a banana or apple.

The ethylene gas made by the regular item will speed up the maturing of the avocado. Stream Free Frozen custards Hold your frozen treats back from streaming onto your hands by setting a little marshmallow at the lower part of the cone past to replenishing in the frozen yogurt.

The marshmallow goes probably as a classy fitting that holds any drained frozen yogurt back from getting down.

terrible Hotcakes as expected Achieve completely round and marginally cooked pancakes by practicing a perfect ketchup flask to control the flapjack megahit.

This hack considers careful part control and accessible round hotcakes predictably. Quick Cool Your Wine Make an effort not to believe that your white wine will chill in the cooler.

All impacts being equivalent, keep frozen grapes in the cooler and drop a couple into your glass of wine.

They'll cool your wine without binding it. Safeguard Against Air pocket Over Spot a provincial spoon across the loftiest mark of a pot of washing water to hold it back from washing over.

The provincial spoon breaks the face tension of the air pockets and holds them inside appropriate cutoff points.

Really bar Eggshells Exactly when a little piece of eggshell falls into your stadium, it will in general be a test to recuperate.

wet down your cutlet, and the eggshell shard will cut to it like witchery. No really confusing fishing sections with a scoop.

Revive Level Bread To return life to old throw sprinkle it gently with water and in this manner toast it on the cookstove for two or three minutes.

The dampness and power will amp the throw making it taste as of late hotted.

The Ice 3D shape Plate Miracle Ice shape plates are versatile kitchen instruments.

Use them to cover new flavors by setting them in every 3D shape and filling them with olive oil painting.

Indurate and store the flavor in olive oil painting for cooking.

No-Disaster area framework for developing Pomegranates Developing pomegranates can be an unkempt preliminary.

Cut the pomegranate down the center and hold it over a stadium, cut side down.

Provide it with several doors with a provincial spoon, and the seeds will fall into the stadium, leaving the substance.

The Shocking Corn Trick husking slime can be a tasteless issue.
Microwave the muck in its cover for 3-4 sparkles, and when it's done, the case will slide off really, leaving you with impeccably cooked antiquated slime.

Dial In the Ideal Rice food rice can every so often be very great, sporadically not super great, yet it needn't bother with to be.

utilize the" 123" extent for dreadful delicate rice no matter what. That is one segment rice, two areas water, and three segments self control.

" Kitchen Hacks and Tips" is your culinary substitute approach to getting ready and amusing arranging.

These wise misdirects and vigilant simple courses will streamline your time in the kitchen, allowing you to focus on the enjoyment of making tasty blowouts and uncommon dishes.

Whether you are a definitively arranged epicure trained professional or basically starting your culinary journey, these hacks will change your kitchen experience into bone
that is finished, fun, and significantly satisfying.

2. Productive Methodology and Culinary Simple Courses:

Productive Methodology and Culinary Simple Courses cuisine More efficiently. In the realm of cuisine, time is constantly of the essence.

We as a whole carry on with enthralled subsistence, and keeping in mind that we need to appreciate tasteful hand drafted feasts, we do not inescapably in every case have hours to spend in the kitchen.

That's where" Effective ways and Culinary Simple Courses" come as an integral factor. These insightful styles and easy routes are your pass to cooking more efficiently, while as yet delighting the kinds of a home- prepared feast.

The Strong Sluggish Cooker   Slow cookers are the overlooked yet truly great individualities of complete cuisine.

Toss your seasoning in the first part of the day, set it, and fail to flash back it.
At the point when you get back, you will be eaten with the tempting scent of a fully set regale, fit to be served.

Slow cookers do a commodity amazing with negligible exertion from you.

Prep in Groups   rather than slashing vegetables or marinating flesh   constantly, put down openings for clump arrangement.

Cleave, bones, and part out rudiments for the week. Having them instantly accessible will unnaturally dwindle the time you spend in the kitchen during the weeknights.

Rice Cooker Sorcery   Rice cookers are not only for rice. They can   foam vegetables, cook quinoa, and indeed set up a multifariousness of one- pot feasts.

Embrace the rigidity of your rice cooker to smooth out your cuisine cycle. Grasp distance Container Suppers distance vessel suppers are an exposure.

They include insignificant readiness and negligible remittal.

Simply orchestrate your protein and veggies on a baking distance, season, and pop it in the cookstove.

A tasteful, straightforward regale is set snappily. Pre-Cut Accommodation While new seasonings are brilliant,pre-cut andpre-slashed vegetables can be a nonstop redeemer.

multitudinous supermarkets offer pre-cut yield, and keeping in mind that it could be brought kindly.

Moreover, the accommodation can be worth the trouble on those bustling gloamings.   Put coffers into a Food Processor   A food processor is a kitchen idler.

It can cut, bones, shred, and indeed massage admixture.   With this machine, you can unnaturally hash down your planning time for a large number of dishes.

One- Pot Cautions'   One- pot feasts are a gift to enthralled   culinarians. They bear negligible remittal and   constantly bring about a pleasurable and good supper.

Consider a workshop of art like stew, stew, or risotto, and you will perceive the way a solitary pot can convey a fabulous regale.

Cooler Cordial feasts   cuisine in groups and indurating parts is a phenomenal system for having instant feasts close by.

Whether it's mists, galoshes, or gravies, having a veritably important supplied cooler can be a lifeline. Moment Pot for Speed and Adaptability The Moment Pot has surprised the culinary world, and understandably.

It consolidates the rudiments of colorful kitchen machines, including a pressure cooker, slow cooker, and rice cooker.

A flexible instrument can help you with getting ready dishes fleetly and effectively. cuisine with Extras Embrace the craft of cooking with extras.

For example, the former evening's coddled funk can turn out to be the present funk serving of mixed flora or funk haze.

This decreases food squander as well as workshop on your cuisine cycle. No- Bomb Feast Arranging Feast arranging can save investment over the long haul.

Put away the occasion every week to design your feasts, make a shopping rundown, and indeed pre-pack a portion of your seasoning. Along these lines, you will continuously have a strategy for the week ahead.

Effective systems and culinary simple courses are the keys to cooking more efficiently.

These styles and alternate ways empower you to appreciate delicious natively constructed feasts without the tedious issue.

Whether you are a performing complete, a bustling guardian, or in the middle between, these keen ways to deal with cuisine will help you with enjoying the kinds of home- prepared feasts without the culinary pressure. Bon appétit!

Chapter 11:

A Sensible Kitchen:

The Center of Successful Home Cooking.

In the area of home cooking, the kitchen is the center of your culinary space.

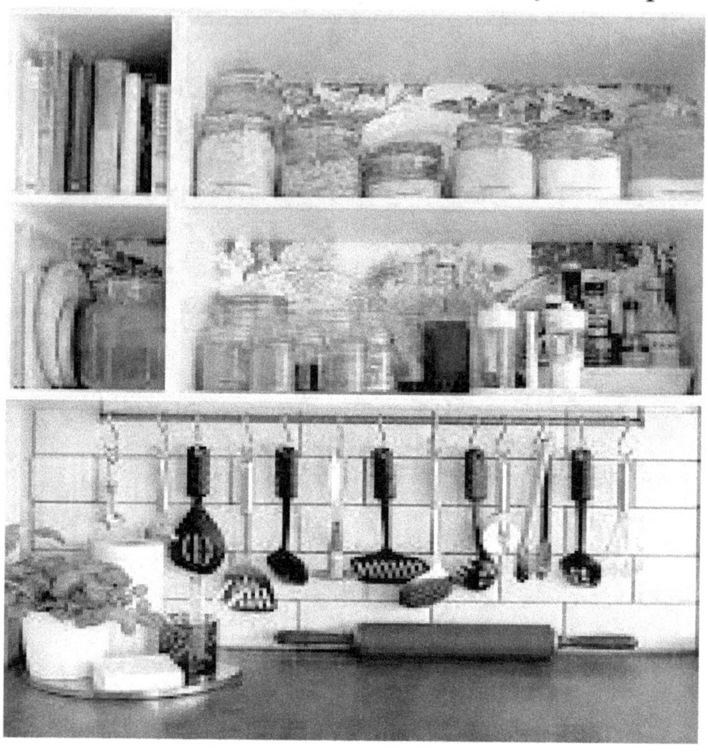

A sensible kitchen is the best approach to achieving successful and beguiling supper preparation.

Whether you're a painstakingly pre-arranged connoisseur master or just starting your cooking interaction, having a productive and helpful kitchen is a particular benefit that can save you time, energy, and make the strategy engaged with cooking more lovely. We ought to explore how to make a kitchen that has capabilities for you.

- Streamlined Workspaces:

Capability in the kitchen starts with a completely inspected design. Ensure your kitchen is composed with clear and portrayed workspaces.

Accumulate similar things, so you're not running starting with one completion of the kitchen then onto the next during supper prep.

Having an alloted district for cutting, slicing, and one something else for cooking deals with your cooking association.

- A Spot for Everything:

A planned kitchen is a sensible kitchen. Put assets into limited game plans like racks, cabinets, and drawers to keep your pots, dishes, utensils, and trimmings productive and actually accessible.

Knowing where everything is saves time and disappointment when you're in the midst of cooking.

- Quality Instruments and Equipment:

Having the right instruments for the gig can essentially streamline your cooking.

Put assets into quality edges, pots, and skillets. A respectable connoisseur expert's sharp edge, for example, can make separating and cutting a breeze, while a non-stick skillet can make your clean up fast and straightforward.

- Capable Machines:

Select kitchen machines that deal with your cooking style. Energy-useful contraptions can save you time, money, and kitchen space.

Mull over placing assets into a food processor to speed up separating, a dishwasher to ease clean up, and a microwave for quick warming.

- Menu Orchestrating:

Plan time to avoid last-minute disorder. Understanding what you will cook and having the trimmings nearby decreases kitchen commotion.

Plan your menus for the week, make a shopping summary, and stick to it. This chips away at the cooking framework as well as help you with staying reasonable for you.

- Keep It Clean:

A sensible kitchen is a flawless kitchen. After each cooking meeting, require two or three minutes to clean up. Put away trimmings, wash dishes, and wipe down surfaces.

An ideal and composed kitchen is inviting and encourages you to cook even more a significant part of the time.

- Moderate System:

A portion of the time hushing up would be ideal. Accepting your kitchen is pouring out done with contraptions and utensils you only from time to time use, consider tidying up.

A moderate kitchen is more direct to regulate and investigate. It also makes it more clear to get to what you truly need.

- Capable Usage of Room:

Increase your kitchen space by using the vertical and even surfaces.

Catches, racks, and resigns can help with keeping utensils, pots, and skillet reachable. Select stackable or settling cookware to save space in your cabinets.

- Tweaked Comfort:

At last, ensure your kitchen is a pleasing and inviting spot to be. Add individual contacts like new flavors on the windowsill, clear dishware, or craftsmanship on the walls. An intriguing kitchen can make cooking a seriously beguiling experience.

- Choice:

Overwhelming a Sensible Kitchen.
A reasonable kitchen is the underpinning of successful home cooking. Composed workspaces, capable limit, quality instruments, and a completely inspected kitchen configuration can streamline your culinary undertakings.

- Menu orchestrating and a moderate technique can moreover deal with your kitchen life.

Remember that your kitchen should be a space that suits your cooking style and rouses your culinary ingenuity.

With a reasonable kitchen, you'll see that the joy of cooking is more open and charming than some other time in ongoing memory.

Along these lines, get in there, get ready something delicious, and value the sorts of home cooking in your as of late improved kitchen.

2. Eco-Accommodating Cooking and Lessening Your Carbon Impression:

Enjoying Maintainable Flavors.
Cooking isn't just about making delectable dinners; it's likewise an amazing chance to settle on eco-accommodating decisions that diminish your carbon impression.

"Eco-Accommodating Cooking and Lessening Your Carbon Impression" is your manual for enjoying manageable flavors while doing whatever it may take to safeguard the planet.

We should investigate how you can cook with a soul and have a constructive outcome on the climate.

- Occasional and Neighborhood Fixings:

One of the least demanding ways of diminishing your carbon impression is to embrace occasional and nearby fixings.

At the point when you pick privately developed produce and fixings in season, you're supporting provincial horticulture and decreasing the fossil fuel byproducts related with significant distance transportation.

- Plant-Based Pleasures:

Integrating plant-based dinners into your cooking advances a solid way of life as well as lessens the ecological effect of creature farming.

Attempt meatless Mondays or investigate the universe of plant-based recipes that praise the assorted and tasty universe of natural products, vegetables, vegetables, and grains.

- Zero-Squander Cooking:

Zero-squander preparation centers around limiting food squander. This can be accomplished by inventively utilizing all pieces of a fixing, for example, using vegetable pieces for natively constructed stocks or sauces. Decreasing food squander is a critical stage in eco-accommodating cooking.

- Practical Fish Determination:

While integrating fish into your dishes, go with feasible decisions by picking species that are not overfished or found utilizing naturally capable strategies.

Search for affirmation marks like MSC (Marine Stewardship Board) to direct your decisions.

- Energy-Proficient Cooking:

Cooking proficiently can save both investments. Use covers on pots and skillet to lessen cooking investment utilization.

Pick energy-proficient machines and cook with the suitable burner size to augment effectiveness.

- Careful Water Use:

Water is a valuable asset, and careful water use is a basic part of eco-accommodating cooking.

Try not to run the tap superfluously and consider reusing pasta water for bubbling vegetables or making soups. Each drop counts.

- Reusable Kitchen Fundamentals:

Decrease squander in your kitchen by utilizing reusable utensils, glass holders, and material napkins.

Kill single-use plastics and settle on reasonable options like bamboo or treated steel.

- Reusing and Fertilizing the soil.

Set up a reusing and fertilizing the soil framework in your kitchen. Appropriately reusing materials and fertilizing the soil food waste can essentially lessen how much waste is shipped off landfills.

- Supporting Practical Brands:

While choosing bundled fixings, support marks that focus on maintainability and eco-accommodating practices.

Search for eco-names and affirmations, like USDA Natural or Fair Exchange, to guarantee you're settling on capable decisions.

- Feast Anticipating Decreased Food Squander:

Feast arranging isn't just a life hack; it likewise decreases food squander. At the point when you plan your dinners, you can purchase just what you really want, and you're more averse to allow fixings to go to squander.

- Diminish and Reuse Extras:

Rather than discarding extras, get inventive and transform them into new dishes.

For instance, the previously cooked vegetables can turn out to be the present frittata.

Diminishing food squander is a tasty method for adding to eco-accommodating cooking.

Conclusion:

- Enjoying Reasonable Flavors:

"Eco-Accommodating Cooking and Diminishing Your Carbon Impression" is an excursion that permits you to relish delectable flavors while pursuing eco-cognizant decisions.

By embracing occasional and nearby fixings, taking on plant-based dinners, and rehearsing zero-squander cooking, you can limit your natural effect. Practical fish, energy-productive cooking, and water care further add to a greener kitchen.

Reusable kitchen fundamentals, reusing, and treating the soil are basic to a more manageable way of life.

Supporting maintainable brands, rehearsing dinner arranging, and tracking down imaginative ways of decreasing and reuse extras complete the recipe for eco-accommodating cooking.

These means decrease your carbon impression as well as energize a better, more capable way to deal with food. By enjoying manageable flavors, you're feeding your body as well as the planet, each luscious dinner in turn.

3. Aware Eating and Food Decisions:

Supporting Body and Psyche.
Food isn't just food; an amazing asset can influence your wellbeing, prosperity, and the climate.

"Discerning Eating and Food Decisions" is your door to the extraordinary universe of careful utilization, where each chomp turns into a chance to sustain your body as well as your brain and the planet.

We should investigate how you can embrace perceptive eating to go with educated and capable food choices.

- Cognizant Fixing Choice:

Insightful eating begins with the fixings you pick. Be aware of the beginning, quality, and medical advantages of your food.

Pick entire, natural fixings, and select natural or economically obtained choices whenever the situation allows.

By understanding what's on your plate, you engage yourself to settle on informed decisions that line up with your qualities.

- Perusing Marks with Expectation:

Pause for a minute to peruse food marks, and not only for carbohydrate contents. Search for buried added substances, additives, and fake fixings.

Get to know the fixings you need to stay away from, for example, high fructose corn syrup, fake tones, and hydrogenated oils. This information will direct you toward better other options.

- Segment Control with Mindfulness:

Practice segment control to forestall gorging and food squander. Focus on your body's yearning and totality signs.

Appreciate each chomp, and take as much time as is needed to partake in the flavors. By standing by listening to your body, you can keep a solid relationship with food.

- Cooking with Reason:

At the point when you set up your feasts, do as such with aim. Cooking at home permits you to control what goes into your food, guaranteeing that you're sustaining your body with healthy fixings.

Think about attempting new recipes and cooking procedures to extend your culinary skylines.

- Diminishing Food Squander:

Be aware of the food you squander. Plan your dinners, use extras imaginatively, and store food appropriately to expand its newness.

By decreasing food squander, you set aside cash as well as add to a more reasonable food framework.

- Careful Food Obtaining:

Support neighborhood ranchers and feasible food makers. Visit ranchers' business sectors and pick food varieties that are in season.

Obtaining locally diminishes the carbon impression related with significant distance transportation and supports your local area.

- Supportable Fish Decisions:

While eating fish, go with economical decisions by alluding to assets like the Fish Watch program.

Keep away from species that are overfished or found utilizing damaging practices. Your decisions can assist with safeguarding our seas and sea-going environments.

- Offset Diet with Healthful Mindfulness:

Make progress toward a decent eating regimen that meets your nourishing necessities.

Know about your dietary prerequisites, and go for the gold of food varieties to guarantee you get many supplements. Incorporate a lot of organic products, vegetables, entire grains, lean proteins, and solid fats in your eating regimen.

- Careful Eating Practices:

Practice careful eating by dispensing with interruptions during feasts. Set aside your gadgets, plunk down, and spotlight on the tactile experience of eating. Relish the surfaces, flavors, and smells.

Careful eating improves your enthusiasm for food as well as advances a better relationship with it.

- Developing Appreciation:

Offer thanks for the food you eat. Perceive the work and assets that went into delivering your feasts. By cultivating a feeling of appreciation for your food, you foster a more profound association with the food it gives.

- Decision: A Supporting Excursion.

"Conscious Eating and Food Decisions" is an extraordinary excursion that supports your body as well as your psyche and the planet.

By being aware of fixing determination, understanding marks, rehearsing segment control, and cooking with a goal, you pursue educated and dependable food choices.

Decreasing food squander, supporting nearby and maintainable obtaining, and embracing a decent eating routine add to a better and more manageable way of life.

Reasonable fish decisions, careful eating rehearsals, and developing appreciation for your dinners extend your association with the food you devour.

With insightful eating, each nibble turns into a chance to pursue decisions that line up with your qualities and add to a better, more cognizant, and really sustaining life.

Chapter 12:

1. The Recipe for Brave Home Cooking:

In the domain of home cooking, culinary certainty is the mysterious fixing that raises your dishes from normal to remarkable.

The Recipe for Brave Home Cooking

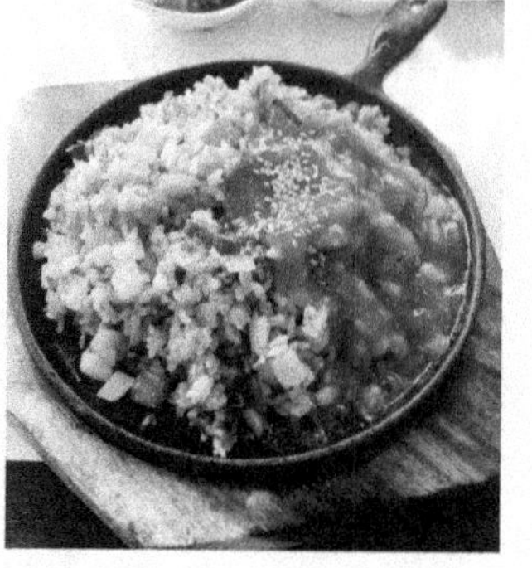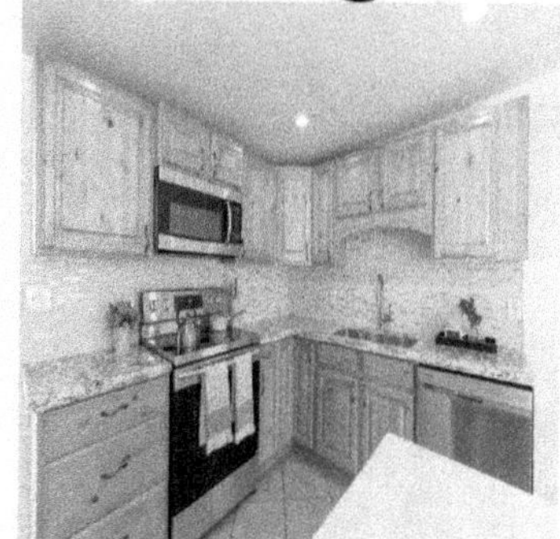

It's the confirmation that you can overcome any recipe, tackle new fixings, and make culinary show-stoppers with energy.

"Culinary Certainty: The Recipe for Valiant Home Cooking" is your manual for becoming the best at cooking with relentless self-assuredness. How about we dig into the universe of culinary sureness and find the keys to culinary achievement.

- Grasping the Essentials:

Culinary sureness begins with grasping the nuts and bolts. Get to know cooking strategies, blade abilities, and fixing profiles.

The more you know, the more engaged you'll feel in the kitchen. Dominating the basics resembles building a strong starting point for your culinary undertakings.

- Embrace Experimentation:

Culinary victory frequently rises out of the remains of kitchen disappointments.

Feel free to commit errors and gain from them. Each overcooked dish, under-prepared feast, or fallen soufflé is an important illustration that will add to your culinary development.

Embrace the course of experimentation, and recall that even prepared culinary specialists experience disasters.

- Get to know New Fixings:

Culinary certainty flourishes when you set out to investigate an unknown culinary area.

Be available to attempt new fixings, flavors, and flavors. Explore different avenues regarding extraordinary natural products, new vegetables, and one of a kind grains. By widening your fixing range, you grow your culinary skylines.

- Embrace Imagination and Variation:

Recipes are rules, not inflexible guidelines. Culinary sureness welcomes you to be imaginative and versatile.

Go ahead and change recipes to suit your taste, or substitute fixings when essential. Cooking turns into a craftsmanship when you put your own touch on each dish.

- Become amazing at Impromptu creation:

Culinary certainty sparkles when you can prepare a dinner from anything that fixings you have close by.

Be the maestro of kitchen impromptu creation. Figuring out how to make dishes from miscellaneous items in your storeroom or refrigerator is an expertise that will work well for you in any culinary circumstance.

- Botches Are Learning Amazing open doors:

In the kitchen, there are no disappointments, just learning potential open doors. On the off chance that a dish doesn't turn out true to form, cheer up.

All things being equal, take apart what turned out badly and consider how to work on it sometime later. It's all important for the excursion toward culinary greatness.

- Consistency Is Vital:

To develop culinary assurance, practice is fundamental. Cook consistently to fabricate your certainty and abilities.

The more you cook, the more recognizable and agreeable you become in the kitchen. The outcome is reliably amazing dishes that mirror your developing certainty.

- Cook with Instinct:

Culinary bosses depend on instinct. As you progress, you'll foster a sharp feeling of taste and timing.

You'll know when a dish needs a touch of salt or a crush of lemon. Pay attention to your gut feelings and let your faculties guide you in the culinary creation process.

- Look for Motivation All over the place:

Motivation for culinary assurance can be found in cookbooks, food web journals, cafés, and, surprisingly, your #1 family recipes.

Investigate new foods, attempt imaginative cooking methods, and seek constantly motivation from the culinary world around you.

- Partake in the Excursion:

Ultimately, make sure to partake in the excursion of culinary revelation. Each dinner you plan is a chance for development, innovativeness, and fulfillment.

Culinary conviction isn't just about the final product; it's about the delight of cooking and the feeling of achievement that accompanies it.

"Culinary Certainty: The Recipe for Dauntless Home Cooking" is your own guide to turning into a bold and talented home gourmet expert.

Figuring out the essentials, embracing experimentation, and getting to know new fixings are the venturing stones to progress.

Dominating inventiveness, act of spontaneity, and the specialty of gaining from botches changes you into a culinary virtuoso.

With each dish you set up, your culinary certainty will take off, and your kitchen will turn into the stage for your culinary magnum opuses.

Embrace the excursion, relish the cycle, and partake in the heavenly products of your recently discovered culinary certainty.

2. Obtaining Expert in the Kitchen:

Your Way to Culinary Dominance
The kitchen, with its sizzling skillet and fragrant flavors, can be a position of imagination and strengthening.

Gaining expertise in the kitchen is tied in with holding onto control, excelling at cooking, and making dishes that leave your friends and family awestruck.

It's an excursion of self-disclosure and gastronomic greatness. Thus, how about we leave this culinary experience and investigate how you can turn into the expert of your kitchen space.

1. Information is Your Power Source

Culinary power begins with information. Jump into cookbooks, cooking shows, and online assets to grow your culinary insight. Grasp the procedures, fixings, and flavor blends that raise your dishes. The more you know, the more certainty you'll acquire.

2. Ace the Fundamentals

Prior to overcoming complex recipes, ace the basics. Master blade abilities, practice different cooking strategies, and grasp the study of baking. A certain culinary expert has areas of strength for an in the nuts and bolts.

3. Put forth Aggressive Objectives

Culinary authority blossoms with laying out and accomplishing aggressive culinary objectives. Challenge yourself with new cooking styles, strategies, or dishes. Your culinary excursion is characterized by the objectives you set, giving an internal compass and accomplishment.

4. Coordinate Your Kitchen Realm

An efficient kitchen is the realm of a sure cook. Organize your utensils, fixings, and hardware such that it sounds good to you. A messiness free and coordinated kitchen advances productivity and lessens pressure.

5. Plan Your Culinary Mission

Plan your feasts like an essential commandant. From weeknight suppers to extraordinary events, a thoroughly examined dinner plan guarantees you have every one of the important fixings, gear, and time to execute your culinary vision with accuracy.

6. Involved Experience Matters

The more you practice, the greater power you aggregate. Continuous cooking meetings permit you to try different things with new procedures, fixings, and styles.

Each culinary undertaking adds to your ability and extends your association with the specialty of cooking.

7. Ace the Ensemble of Flavors

Culinary authority is exemplified by your capacity to blend flavors. Try different things with flavors, spices, and different cooking strategies to make an orchestra of tastes that have an enduring effect on your sense of taste.

8. Adjust and Beat Difficulties

A certain gourmet specialist knows how to adjust and ad lib when confronted with difficulties.

Whether it's a lacking piece or an unexpected disaster, your capacity to think and react quickly and settle culinary riddles is the sign of power.

9. Share Your Culinary Victories

Try not to keep your culinary victories stowed away. Share your dishes with loved ones and look for input.

Sharing your manifestations isn't simply an opportunity to exhibit your mastery yet in addition a chance to refine your culinary abilities.

10. Embrace the Innovative Odyssey

Recollect that the kitchen is your material, and your dishes are your masterpieces.
Embrace the imaginative odyssey that cooking offers. Expert in the kitchen isn't just about following recipes; it's tied in with communicating your novel style and making dishes that mirror your culinary enthusiasm.

Securing expertise in the kitchen is a continuous experience that joins information, ability, and imagination.

It's tied in with dominating the fundamentals, putting forth objectives, arranging your kitchen, arranging dinners, and acquiring active experience.

The capacity to adjust flavors, adjust to difficulties, and offer your manifestations with others means your development as a certain culinary expert.

As you embrace this culinary excursion, you'll find that being an expert in the kitchen isn't just about cooking; about making workmanship amuses the faculties and makes a permanent imprint on the palates of the people who appreciate your culinary magnum opuses.

Thus, leave on your way to culinary authority with certainty and enthusiasm, and let the kitchen become your material for gastronomic brightness.

3. Testing and Idealizing Your Recipes:

The excursion of a home cook is a ceaseless journey for culinary greatness. It's a way loaded up with trial and error, disclosure, and an intermittent slip up.

Testing and culminating your recipes is the substance of this experience, where you change crude fixings into flavorful manifestations.

This interaction is much the same as culinary speculative chemistry, and it's the manner by which you can genuinely make a recipe your own.

We should investigate the specialty of testing and consummating your culinary manifestations.

- The Primary Endeavor:

Each culinary work of art starts with a first endeavor. At the point when you're anxious to attempt another recipe, follow it near figure out the essentials.

This underlying exertion is your material; it's where you establish the groundwork for the dish you mean to make.

Try not to be discouraged by blemishes at this stage; they are important for the inventive strategy.

- Embrace Variety:

The enchantment of consummating a recipe frequently lies in embracing variety. Change the recipe in unobtrusive ways, modifying fixings, extents, or cooking techniques to suit your taste. Take notes on what you change, and see how these alterations impact the result.

- Taste, Taste, Taste:

Testing and idealizing a recipe requires your taste buds to be your most noteworthy pundits.

Routinely taste your dish as it develops. This will assist you with recognizing subtleties, grasp the equilibrium of flavors, and make the essential changes.

- Record Your Excursion:

Keep a culinary diary or computerized notes as you test. Record each change you make and its impact on the dish.

This record will act as your aide, permitting you to backtrack your means when you find that brilliant proportion of fixings and strategies.

- Persistence is an Uprightness:

Idealizing a recipe can be a tedious interaction, and persistence is fundamental.

It might take various endeavors to arrive at the ideal outcome, yet each try carries you one bit nearer to culinary flawlessness.

- Look for Criticism:

Feel free to do your culinary tests with loved ones. Their criticism can give significant bits of knowledge and alternate points of view on your dishes. A subsequent assessment might uncover flavors or surfaces you've missed.

- Fixing Quality Matters

The nature of fixings can significantly affect the result of your dishes. Put resources into the best quality fixings you can manage, as they can raise your recipes higher than ever. New, top notch fixings are much of the time the way flawlessly.

- Keep a Feeling of Experience:

While testing and idealizing recipes is an organized interaction, keep a feeling of experience.

Don't hesitate for even a moment to be unpredictable, to defy the norms, or to add your unique wind to an exemplary recipe.

The absolute most eminent dishes were made when cooks thought for even a second to be gutsy.

- Observe Your Victories:

With every emphasis, you're nearer to your culinary objective. Praise the victories en route, paying little heed to how little they might appear.

Perceive that each work carries you nearer to becoming amazing at culinary speculative chemistry.

- A Recipe that Communicates in Your Language:

Eventually, the recipe you wonderful is as of now not simply a bunch of guidelines; it's a piece of you.

It communicates in your language, mirrors your culinary excursion, and epitomizes your one of a kind flavor inclinations. Culminating a recipe resembles making a piece of craftsmanship; it's a statement of your innovativeness and enthusiasm.

Testing and consummating your recipes is where the sorcery occurs in the realm of home cooking. It's an excursion of investigation, trial and error, and development.

With each endeavor, you're one bit nearer to culinary authority, and your recipes develop into flavorful show-stoppers that convey your unmistakable culinary character.

In this way, embrace the cycle, appreciate the flavors, and partake in the change from crude fixings to culinary show-stoppers that are genuinely your own.

Conclusion:

- **The Excursion Ahead:**

Cooking Shrewd and Eating Great for a Lifetime.
As we finish up our culinary journey through the universe of "Cook Shrewd, Eat Well," now is the right time to ponder the surprising excursion we've set out on.

This isn't simply a cookbook; it's a manual for a long period of careful and flavorful eating. We've covered the fundamentals of cooking, from dominating kitchen nuts and bolts to investigating worldwide flavors.

We've embraced maintainability and cognizant eating, and we've figured out how to get expert in the kitchen. Presently, we should look forward to the deep rooted excursion of cooking brilliantly and eating great.

- A Maintainable Culinary Way of life:

One of the persevering through illustrations of this culinary investigation is the significance of maintainability.

By picking occasional, nearby fixings and embracing eco-accommodating cooking rehearses, you're feeding your body as well as adding to a better planet.

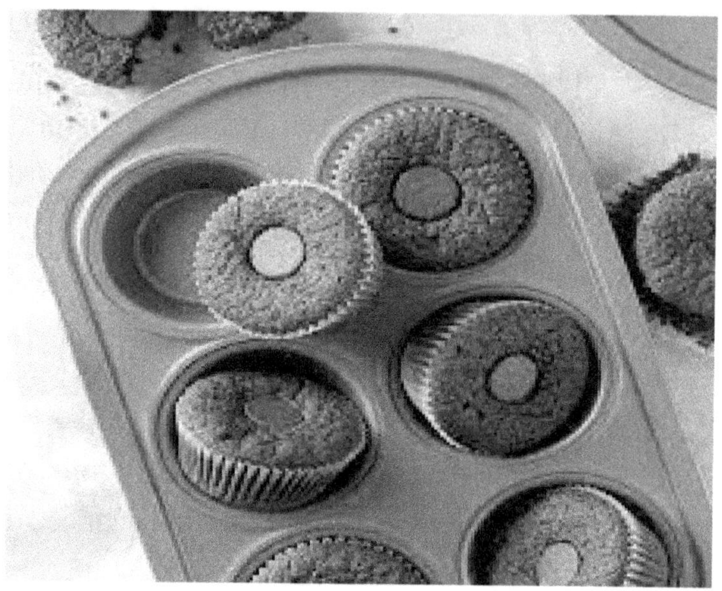

Economical decisions aren't simply a pattern; they're a lifestyle that can help you and people in the future.

- Culinary Certainty: Your Own Superpower:

Obtaining expertise in the kitchen is something other than dominating recipes; it's tied in with building culinary certainty. It's the conviction that you can make, adjust, and make do with fixings and procedures.

This certainty engages you to try and make dishes that mirror your remarkable style, charming the individuals who appreciate your manifestations.

- Careful and Mindful Eating:

Perceptive eating is tied in with pursuing educated and mindful food decisions. It's a pledge to figuring out fixings, understanding marks, and supporting neighborhood and maintainable sources.

By taking on a careful way to deal with food, you're taking care of your body, yet additionally feeding your prosperity and supporting a better food framework.

- The Craft of Recipe Testing and Flawlessness:

Culminating a recipe is a demonstration of your devotion and innovativeness. It's an excursion of experimentation, of refining your culinary vision.

Each dish you wonderful turns into a work of art, an impression of your developing abilities and taste inclinations. An update cooking is a workmanship, a science, and a beautiful source of both pain and joy.

- The Continuous Culinary Odyssey:

As you proceed with your culinary excursion, recall that the kitchen is your material, and every dinner is a chance to make, find, and appreciate.

You're not simply cooking; you're making culinary encounters that give pleasure, sustenance, and pride.

- A Long period of Clever Cooking and Careful Eating:

Cooking shrewd and eating great isn't an objective; it's a long lasting undertaking. It's tied in with relishing the excursion, continually learning, and developing your culinary abilities.

It's tied in with praising the heavenly flavors and fixings accessible to you, whether in your nearby market or on a worldwide scale.

Conclusion:

- The Culinary Heritage You Leave:

"Cook Shrewd, Eat Well" is in excess of a cookbook; it's a culinary heritage. It's a promise to economical living, culinary certainty, cognizant eating, and the specialty of recipe flawlessness.

It's a demonstration of your affection for good food and your devotion to making a better and more tasty world.

As you proceed with your excursion, remember the delight of imparting your culinary manifestations to friends and family.

Dinners arranged with care and innovativeness have the ability to fortify connections and make enduring recollections. Your culinary heritage isn't just about the dishes you awesome; it's about the minutes you make around the table.

In this way, continue investigating new cooking styles, attempting new fixings, and embracing the culinary experiences that look for you.

Cooking shrewd and eating great isn't just about today; it's about a long period of tasty, careful, and manageable living.

As you set out on this culinary odyssey, may your kitchen be loaded up with the smell of delectable manifestations, and may your heart be warmed by the delight of imparting them to those you love. Bon appétit!